Beyond the Baby Blues

Beyond the Baby Blues

Anxiety and Depression During and After Pregnancy

Rebecca Fox Starr

ROWMAN & LITTLEFIELD
Lanham • Boulder • New York • London

Published by Rowman & Littlefield
A wholly owned subsidiary of The Rowman & Littlefield Publishing Group, Inc.
4501 Forbes Boulevard, Suite 200, Lanham, Maryland 20706
www.rowman.com

Unit A, Whitacre Mews, 26-34 Stannary Street, London SE11 4AB

British Library Cataloguing in Publication Information Available

Library of Congress Cataloging-in-Publication Data
Names: Fox Starr, Rebecca, 1985– author.
Title: Beyond the baby blues : anxiety and depression during and after
  pregnancy / Rebecca Fox Starr.
Description: Lanham : Rowman & Littlefield, [2018] | Includes bibliographical
  references and index.
Identifiers: LCCN 2017023086 (print) | LCCN 2017024659 (ebook) |
  ISBN 9781442273917 (electronic) | ISBN 9781442273900 (cloth : alk. paper)
Subjects: LCSH: Postpartum depression. | Postpartum depression—Treatment.
Classification: LCC RG852 (ebook) | LCC RG852 .F69 2018 (print) |
  DDC 618.7/6—dc23
LC record available at https://lccn.loc.gov/2017023086

Printed in the United States of America

For my Kenny:
For seeing the light go out in my eyes,
and then for bringing it back.

Contents

Acknowledgments

I am supremely grateful to many people for helping to make this—my dream—into a reality. As I often say, my tribe is the best tribe; and this book, aimed at helping women, caregivers, and members of the healthcare community, is my cherished labor of love.

Thank you to my agent, the amazing and talented Renée C. Fountain, president of Gandolfo Helin & Fountain Literary Management agency. Renée, you believed in me and in this project, even with all of the twists, turns, curveballs, changes, and obstacles that have been thrown our way. You recognized my passion and supported me through every step of this journey, and I will be eternally grateful for your expertise, patience, and strength. Thank you to the rest of the team at Gandolfo Helin & Fountain for being an incredibly supportive community of writers, artists, and rabble-rousers.

Many thanks to the Rowman & Littlefield team. A huge thanks to my editor, Suzanne Staszak-Silva. Suzanne, you gave me the greatest gift with just one word: "yes." I am so grateful that you turned this project into the bold, unique text that it is today, one that is packed with actionable advice about prenatal distress, setting us apart in this expansive industry. I know that, because of you, we will help to save other women from the pain that I endured. Thank you also to my production editor, Patricia Stevenson, for your kindness, patience, enthusiasm, and help.

Thank you to Dr. Judith Beck, who has supported me since day one of this project, sending me articles, giving me support, and introducing me to

Dr. Amy Wenzel. Dr. Beck, you are a force of nature. And to Dr. Wenzel: I literally could not have done this without you. It has been an honor laughing, crying, and writing with you. You are a true expert in your field and we are so lucky to have your wisdom, experience, and case studies in this book. Thank you for your time, transparency, and talent.

Thank you to Mike Greenspoon, creative director of Brand Revive, for giving me a logo, an identity, and a website that I am proud to call my own. Thank you to Kimberly Ettinger, president of Pearl Communications, for supporting me every step of the way, helping me with my public relations goals, and teaching me how to properly use a hashtag.

I would not be here today if it were not for the *Mommy, Ever After* online support group, nicknamed #teamMEA. Ladies, you are the heart and soul of why I write. Thank you for sharing your darkest moments with me, for contributing to this project, and for giving us a collective voice. You are my "why." We have been through some hard times, as a group, but never, ever, ever stop fighting. You are worth it. You deserve this. This book is for you.

I am so grateful for my treatment team. Thank you for holding my hand when I've needed warmth, pushing me when I've needed tough love, and never judging me for being who I am. I literally would not be here today without you.

And now, I say thank you to my family, both by chance and by choice. You have supported me as a writer—and as a human—in more ways than I could ever name. Mom and Dad, you have instilled in me the value of helping others. That is why I am able to write the things that other people are afraid to put on paper. Thank you for holding my hand through the darkest of days and for never giving up on me or on this project. You have taught me about empathy, compassion, and unconditional love; you have made me into the parent that I am today. Emily, you inspire me with your work ethic, determination, and poise and I am so proud that you are my little sister. Speaking of sisters, thank you to my sisters of the soul. Each one of you holds a special place in my life, in my story, and in my heart. You know who you are. I love you ever so much.

Dear Kenny, you are my hero. We may have been to hell and back, but thankfully we can just look at it as another (short) trip on our long list of adventures together. You are my rock and my rock star. I feel blessed, each and every day, that I was wise enough at twenty years old to say "yes" to a date with the "bad boy" from around the corner. You never cease to amaze me with your strength, never stop stunning me with your compassion, and you have never given up on us, even in our darkest days. I will love you forever and I will like you for always.

Annabelle Lily and Alexander Beau: this is for you. Not just this book, but everything. Every word I write is for you two, as you make my heart beat, my soul sing, and my life worth living. There is no greater title on earth than being "Belle and Beau's Mommy," as you are extraordinary people, whom I am so proud to call mine. Thank you for giving me endless material, an infinite amount of kisses, and a life that is filled with magic. You are my happily ever after.

Introduction

Emergency rooms 3 and 4 were connected, but separated by a thin curtain that could be opened in order to create a makeshift suite. In room 4, in a stretcher that appeared humongous, lay my son, three days shy of being two months old. He was hooked up to an IV, had an oxygen monitor taped to his tiny toe, and was receiving a constant stream of oxygen through a tube in his nose. In room 3, I lay, dizzy and disoriented, chained to an IV pole and receiving my third bag of fluids. A nurse handed me a yellow pill. Potassium. She told me that I was deficient and to swallow.

"Do you feel safe?" she asked. I did not. I tugged at the arm of my sweater, reflexively, to make sure that the scratches on my arm were not visible.

We were in a suite in the emergency room of a hospital. He and I were together, but still so far apart, as we were each confined to our beds. We were ailing. We were both being poked and tested and medicated. We both needed help.

Part I
A HAPPY STORY

1

❖ ❖

First Comes Love

A Pregnant Paws and Other Crazy Tales

O nce upon a time, in the suburbs of Philadelphia, I met and married the boy who grew up around the corner. And we lived . . . well, we lived through many things. But I should back up.

My happy story began long before I met my husband, Kenny, but in order to tell this story I am going to start in March 2006, when I cut him off with my car.

Though we had both gone away for college, in 2006, Kenny and I found ourselves back home, in the town where we had grown up. We were raised in a neighborhood that was a mecca for young families: ten streets, each named for a Revolutionary War general, surrounding General Wayne Park. I lived at 519 Mercer Road until I was ten years old. Kenny was raised at 518 Monroe Road. We grew up one street apart.

Despite our nearly four-year age difference, we share so many of the same childhood memories: the same mailman, the same ice cream truck, the same neighbors and babysitters, the same hours spent in the park that we could each see from our own bedroom window. We sat on the same merry-go-round so many times as children that it would be impossible to count.

And, like every good, neurotic child from "The Main Line," we saw the same therapist. I went to cope with my beloved grandmother's death, and Kenny went during his parents' divorce. The stuff of fairy tales.

Though we had attended the same school since preschool, we never became friends, nor did we connect until that early spring in 2006 when we each found ourselves back in the burbs, looking for something. Someone, really.

Thanks to a brief dip in the pool of online dating, some close mutual friends, and serendipity, as it were, I became connected to a young man named Kenny Starr. When I first saw his name appear on my computer screen, it took a moment for me to place him.

Kenny Starr? This kid had been a senior when I was a freshman in high school. We had taken the same bus. He had a reputation.

So, within a few seconds of seeing his name on my laptop, I decided that I most certainly would not be dating him. I canceled my online dating memberships, but Kenny somehow got my screen name. Even when he sent me an incredibly kind first message, I was certain that we were just going to be friends. Though he continued to reach out to me every day, I had no expectations. Except our conversations were amazing. Exciting, different, fun, familiar. We talked, moving from the computer screen to the phone. The first thing that I noticed was his beautiful voice, which I still cannot describe in words, but I think that it is what first made me start to fall in love with him. In those early days, we talked about our lives and shared secrets, and the minutes turned into hours as we talked through the night and into the morning.

Until, one day, I had to cut our conversation short. I had an appointment. I told Kenny that I was going to the allergist. In truth, however, I was going to see my therapist. The aforementioned shared therapist.

Even though we had bonded a great deal over the phone, I wasn't quite ready to tell this guy, a guy whom I'd never really met, that I was going to see a shrink. I was twenty years old and not quite comfortable talking about mental health issues—which, at the time, for me, were limited to a mild case of anxiety with a few irrational fears thrown in—before a first date. And so I told him that we would talk after my allergy appointment, and I went to tell my therapist all about this new, exciting guy.

After my appointment, anxious to go home and finish my conversation with my crush, I pulled out of the therapist's long driveway and cut off a black Volkswagen with my black Toyota. I looked up, and, though it happened so quickly before we each sped away, I saw the face of my crush behind the wheel. Kenny Starr. I had cut off Kenny Starr while pulling out of the driveway to my therapist's office. Horror.

I got a text message within a minute. "Was that you in the black Camry?" he asked.

And so I did the noble, honest, admirable thing: I lied through my teeth.

"Oh, really? That was you? That's so funny. Yeah, so after the allergist I took the long way home and was turning around in a random driveway in Gladwyne! So funny!"

"It is funny," he said, earnestly and innocently. "You actually turned around in the driveway of the shrink I used to see when my parents were separating."

Bless his heart. A day later I came clean; later that week we had our first real date, to which he brought me Rice Krispies Treats instead of the traditional flowers (smart man!), and after he dropped me off that night I called my mom.

"You are going to marry him," she said. And she was right.

From the very beginning we fit together like two puzzle pieces, with an instant level of comfort and support that typically comes with age and time. He said the right things, and not because he had game (he did not) but because he is a good human being. The best.

He always made me feel wanted, and seen, and loved. In those very early days, he would surprise me at my apartment door after a long day apart, just so that we could give each other a kiss good night. He always answered my calls and messages, and when I asked him if he wanted to make plans, he never played games. He invited me into his world with open arms and an even more open heart. And it should be noted that he kept my pantry stocked with an endless supply of Rice Krispies Treats. The good, fancy kind, too.

A few months later, Kenny and I spent our first summer together down at the Jersey Shore. In those days we would sit on the beach for hours on end, watching as the families retreated, lugging their umbrellas, coolers, and kids into minivans, parked tightly on our beach-block street. One summer evening we stayed out later than usual, until we were the only people left on the beach. We sat in beach chairs, tracing our feet in the warm sand, watching the sun retreat into the horizon.

The first weekend we spent "down the shore" (as they say in the glorious Philadelphia suburbs) together was also the first weekend that my husband met my extended family. He was coming into my life at a difficult time for all of us, as we were dealing with the horrible and unexpected illness that was afflicting my uncle. My dad's younger brother, Andy, was battling stage-four metastatic melanoma. It had come out of nowhere. Uncle Andy was forty-three. We were all a little off that summer, but Kenny managed to stay strong for me, offering love and support, even though he was wading through somewhat tumultuous, and definitely new, oceans. So many things became very real that weekend. I remember silently daydreaming about our future, something that seemed so far away, yet so very real. And I had something very important to tell him: our baby's name.

We were not engaged. I was not pregnant. Our daughter would not be born for many more years. But, that day, I knew her name, and I had to get his approval. I remember how nervous I was, drawing graffiti in the sand with my fingers, hoping, with all of my might, that he would say yes to me. Because I was not just asking this man, my new boyfriend, to agree to a future name for our future baby; I was really asking him for a future. To have babies with me. To agree to a family. And to a forever.

That weekend, my husband met and got to bond with the member of my family who would not see the following summer. My Uncle Andy would not be able to dance with us at our wedding or hold up our chuppah. He did not get to swing me around his massive, tattooed arm in a rowdy Horah. He wouldn't be there when our children were born. Although, if I am being totally honest, I believe that he was actually there for all of these moments. He would, however, be the one whom my husband would call, just a few months later, to ask his permission, along with my dad's, for my hand in marriage. And he would be the person for whom our daughter is named. The same name that I had told my husband on the beach that day, during that first summer. Annabelle.

So on that day, years ago, sitting in the sand, as the sun began to fade, Kenny became a member of our family. And as my uncle's life had begun to fade, this family morphed and shifted, undulating like the ocean before us. That summer, Kenny agreed to so much more than a baby name.

He would be there for me, and for all of us, in good times and in bad, in health, and through devastating sickness. He agreed to it all that day. He said yes to our tomorrow, for as long as we both should live.

In 2008 we got married, went on a honeymoon, and bought a house. And after years of being together, we would still stay up until all hours of the night, talking and laughing, just like in our early phone conversations of years past. I would often go to bed with my stomach hurting, because I had been belly laughing so hard. Kenny has always known how to make me laugh.

In 2009, after our first year of marriage, I got the baby bug, and I got it bad. I was ready to get pregnant and to get on it. On. It. After much discussion, and perhaps a bit of nagging, Kenny agreed, pulling me aside during our family's Thanksgiving dinner.

"Maybe next year at Thanksgiving we can say, 'We have something else to be thankful for.' I think that would be very cool," he said.

And, just like that, we were trying. And then, when I didn't get pregnant the very first month, we went from "trying" to "Trying to Conceive," or, as it was often called, "TTC," a distinction that anyone dealing with fertility issues—big or small, short term or permanent—knows well. Some people would call my approach to getting pregnant "impatient"; I am going to go with "impassioned." I had always dreamed of becoming a mother, and once we started to try it could not happen soon enough. After the first few months without success, I started to scour message boards, look for signs of ovulation, and cry. I was the first of my friends to get married and to try to have a baby, and so I had no one in whom to confide who could actually relate. My best friends were fantastic and supportive, but they had no idea what the hell I was talking about when I asked them about egg-white cervical mucus and if they had ever noticed it.

It took eight months, dozens of pee tests, many ultrasounds, a few visits to a specialist (who said that I had no fertility issues whatsoever), and a major dose of chilling the heck out, but in August 2009 I found out that I was pregnant. And not only was I pregnant, but my baby was also due the exact same day that my mom had been due with me: April 18.

If there is such a thing as normal, my pregnancy with my daughter was pretty darn "statistically average." I, however, was not. I was anxious, making sure to do everything "right." And so I was careful not to lift anything heavy, I took my prenatal vitamins religiously, and I avoided deli meat, nitrates, and unpasteurized cheese. Those things would be, to use the aforementioned term, normal for a pregnant woman.

At twenty weeks we had our anatomy scan, during which time an ultrasound technician shows you every part of your growing baby. Though we had originally decided to wait on finding out the sex so that it would be a "surprise," we called an audible while the tech had her wand down between the baby's legs.

"Well, here is her bottom," the tech told us.

"There isn't anything there," said my husband.

"I see three lines," I said, shakily.

I knew what those three lines meant. We were having a girl.

For anyone who says that by finding out the sex of the baby before delivery you are missing out on a great surprise, I am here to say that in that moment, in the small hospital exam room, I felt more surprised, grateful, happy, and emotional than I could have ever imagined. Not one ounce of joy or wonder was taken away by finding out the sex during my scan. My husband and I hugged and cried.

"We get to plan a wedding," I whispered, which is what my mom said when I was born and placed upon her chest.

Finding out that our baby was a girl made things all the more exciting and all the more real, but it also increased my level of stress. She stopped being an unknown and, in my mind, was a person, with a name, and so my fretfulness caused me to take things to a whole new level. One night, I was mistakenly served tonic water instead of club soda. I called the doctor convinced that I had inadvertently poisoned my baby with quinine. Another time I called the obstetrician's emergency line to make sure that the expired bottle of Honest Tea that I had consumed but one third of was not going to cause irreversible damage.

And then there were the Google searches. These included, but were not limited to:

"Baby safe when 25 lb. dog jumps on pregnant belly?"
"Does the sound of a hair dryer scare a fetus in the womb?"
"Do coffee shops ever accidentally serve caffeinated coffee posing as decaf?"

Needless to say, I avoided caffeine (and herbs in tea—and medicine).

And despite my desperate attempt to have control over my pregnancy by following all of the rules, preparing for natural childbirth with hypnosis training, and being a straight-A vessel of life, I ended up with a birth experience that was nothing like I had expected.

I was ready to take on labor like a champ, or so I thought, when my contractions, which I had been having for weeks, started to come at short, regular intervals during my fortieth week of pregnancy.

I went to sleep on a Wednesday night, feeling a strong, tight pulling sensation in my abdomen. Once the pain increased, I started to casually clock them. They were coming every five minutes. Knowing that I would be heading to the hospital the next morning to meet my daughter, I could hardly sleep. "Only one more night to go," I thought. "My dreams will really be coming true."

By morning, I was experiencing "the magic formula" for contractions: they were five minutes apart, they lasted for at least one minute each time, and the episode continued for more than one hour. I had been having intense Braxton Hicks contractions for weeks and weeks, where my entire stomach would tighten up into a crazy, lopsided knot. When this would happen, I was actually happy to be having these practice contractions, because I felt like my uterus would be in good, fighting shape for the big day—the real thing. And, at some point, I was sure they would start to help my dilation/effacement process.

And so, by 8 a.m. on that Thursday morning, I had been having regular, painful contractions every five minutes, lasting more than one minute each, for about ten hours. I called the OBGYN and told him that I was in pain. He told me that he was happy to hear that.

"Come on in!" he said, enthusiastically.

"This had better not be a false alarm. I refuse to be one of those false alarm people!" I told my husband.

"You are so in labor," my husband told me.

"I can't wait to meet you!" I told the baby.

I put some blush on my cheeks, wrangled our dogs, and grabbed our hospital bag, and we were off to meet our baby.

My husband and I had made the mutual decision to have my mom with us in the delivery room. We both wanted to be able to hold her hand, if need be, and I knew she would be able to be strong, even if it got scary. She had been through it, twice, and could be the motivation I needed to stick with my au naturel labor plan. Plus, my husband had previously experienced episodes during which he would be a little queasy. If he went down, I needed a backup.

So we grabbed my mom and off we went.

I felt pretty good walking into the hospital and waddling (stopping every few minutes during contractions) up to labor and delivery.

When the resident came in to examine me, before my obstetrician arrived, we were all surprised to learn that I hadn't progressed at all from my checkup earlier in the week. However, my contractions were strong, long, and regular, so the doctor told me that this was just early labor, and that I'd be in full-blown labor in no time.

The physician told me that she had a "good feeling." So, we waited. And waited. And three hours later, my contractions only intensified.

My OBGYN came in to visit me. I was in tremendous pain and felt tears stinging my eyes. My doctor took one look at me and said, "You're not in real labor. I can tell by looking at your face."

I was in shock. Shock and rage. "What do you mean, 'not in real labor'? Aren't you seeing my contractions on the monitor? Don't you see these tears?"

But, as the nurse told me, in real labor, I wouldn't be able to walk and talk. When that time came, I would just know.

And, just as the doctor had predicted, my exam revealed that I had not progressed at all in those three hours.

I was one centimeter dilated and 50 percent effaced. He assuaged my disappointment by telling me not to worry, that he would most definitely be seeing me in twenty-four to forty-eight hours for the real deal. And . . . they sent me home. When you are forty weeks pregnant, have been on bed rest for six weeks (did I mention that I had to go on bed rest, as I was experiencing some vertigo that made me a "fall risk"? Because that happened), and are swollen, miserable, and desperately impatient and unreasonably anxious, having to waddle out of the hospital without a baby in your arms is not a fun thing.

Plus, I was a little embarrassed. Yes, all signs had pointed to labor, and yes, the doctor himself had told me to come in. And yes, the doctors who had examined me in labor and delivery were sure that I was in labor. But it was not a good feeling, to add to the other not good feelings happening south of the border.

The next morning came and went. I bounced on my big, silver gym ball. I pressed all of the acupressure points that I knew how to find. I ate approximately nine whole pineapples. I could still walk and could still talk, and I told myself that I would not be going back into labor and delivery until it was really, truly, beyond a shadow of a doubt time to give birth. I would hold out as long as posssssssssssssssssible, so that by the time I arrived, all that I would have to do was to push. Maybe once or twice.

But, in reality, at the time, I was in agony. Not only had I not slept in two nights, but I was also having strong contractions every few minutes, and, worse than that, I was in a horrible state of unknowing.

In order to distract me, my mom took me out on a shopping trip, and after a day of walking and contracting I sat down on my bed, put my feet up, and looked at the clock. It was four o'clock on Friday afternoon. I stretched my legs and leaned my head back, and then, suddenly, there was water.

There was no big gush of water, but I felt water pour out from me, and I had not peed myself. This was not the "buckets" that had been described by friends, my doctor, and my labor class when people spoke of the water breaking. It was nothing like what they show in the movies. But I knew that it was something. And though it was a small amount, it continued.

Once again, I called the special emergency-after-hours line for my obstetrician's office and spoke to the nurse.

"Your water broke. Your membranes are ruptured. We need to be very careful now. Come on in. And hurry."

Finally, the time had come. I could scarcely believe that it was actually happening. I had heard that a water breaking was something that happened to women in only about 10 percent of pregnancies, so I had doubted strongly that I would ever find myself in that select group. But, sure enough, water, water everywhere. Back to the hospital I went.

Once again we drove to my parents' house, once again we dropped off my dogs, once again I reminded my dad to give them "tons" of extra love and kisses, and once again I walked (yes, I could still walk, but this time I had a broken water . . .) into the hospital, rode the excruciatingly long elevator ride up to the labor and delivery unit, and planted myself on the hospital bed. I was in for the long haul. Once again, a resident came in to do my examination. And, once again, she looked at me, sheepishly, and told me that I would not like what she had to say.

According to my internal examination, I was one centimeter dilated and 50 percent effaced.

"Um, no. That is actually not possible. I'm sorry, but you must be mistaken. Or crazy. You're crazy! I must have progressed since yesterday. I have been contracting every three minutes for forty-eight hours. My water broke!"

I cannot say with full confidence and a clear memory that this was my exact quote, but I know that I said some, if not a variation, of all of those things, and maybe more. And there were tears. I may even have thrown some things. Expletives, at the very least.

I think the young doctor shrugged, apathetically. And so, once again, they had me wait, while running tests to determine what was going on with my stubborn cervix. At one point, my blood pressure went up, which was because I was upset and scared, and that's what happens when people are in distress.

I asked the resident, "I know that my blood pressure just got high, but am I OK?" She just looked at me and shook her head, slowly, from side to side.

Predictably, I was not, in fact, OK. I waited more, they tested more, and, finally, the resident came back in to tell me that no, my water had not, in fact, broken.

I was incredulous. There had been water. And although not in copious amounts, there was enough. I had felt it pour out of me, out of nowhere. I had felt it continue to leak. And because we are getting truly intimate here, I will share that it was clear and it happened several times. The physician could not explain it. She just said that my water had not broken and that I had not dilated or effaced any more. I was sent home, again.

By that point, I stormed and stomped (still waddling) out of the hospital, determined that my baby would just live in me forever, growing up in my womb, graduating from high school, and then college, from inside my bulging belly. It would never end.

I went to bed that Friday night feeling hopeless.

I woke up the next day, a nice Saturday morning, feeling desperate, but also a little concerned. My baby was being a little quiet. It's not that I wasn't feeling her move at all; I was. Just not as much, and not the same way. I was a little freaked out, but I recalled an old wives' tale out there that claims that a baby slows down and grows quiet the day before a woman goes into labor. I kept this kernel in the back of my mind but couldn't quell the butterflies that were flying around the quieter baby in my belly.

I spent the day walking around, bouncing, fretting, and whining, and I went for a pedicure. At the nail salon, I happened to be seated next to a nice, young doctor who worked at the hospital where I would be delivering.

She was a general practitioner, not an OBGYN, but that did not stop me from peppering her with anxious questions. I asked her if it was normal that my baby was being significantly more quiet. I kept using the word "quiet," because I could not think of a more appropriate or descriptive word to describe what I was feeling. Or, I should say, what I was not feeling.

The kind doctor told me that I should be feeling the baby moving throughout the day, and that if I still hadn't felt much in a few hours, I should be sure to call the doctor's office. The emergency line. We exchanged smiles, and I got her business card and held on to it, along with the worry that was in my heart.

Something just didn't feel right.

There is a very common belief that a mother has some sort of inexplicable, possibly divine, intuition. Well, this was it. It was noon and I decided to take another walk, this time around an outdoor shopping area. I could barely move by this point in the day, but I was determined to stay on my feet in the hopes that gravity would work its magic.

My husband and I strolled, but even as I walked and contracted, I couldn't push away the anxious feeling that was rising inside of me. I was feeling my baby move occasionally, but it was just different.

I could write the whole story now about the next thing that happened that day—the thing that started an avalanche of events that are so unbelievable that I would absolutely be incredulous had I not lived through this myself. If you recall, I used to see a therapist for mild anxiety and some fears, which included separation anxiety. My phobias were my mind's way of preparing me for the worst: loss. So, when I was hobbling around the shopping pavilion and saw my phone light up with my mom's name, I answered, expecting to complain to her about my abject agony, but she cut me off.

"Bex, something happened. There's been an accident," she said. And then my world stopped. I, like my baby, went silent. The news was this: My mom's sister, my dear aunt, had been trying to park her large SUV in an underground garage in downtown Philadelphia, but it would not fit without moving a traffic cone. When she got out to move the cone to make room for her truck, the vehicle, not properly placed in the "park" position, ran over her. She was alive, but one side of her small body had been completely crushed.

This news distracted me. I do not know how I got home from the shopping center that afternoon, but the next thing I remember was choking down a dinner of a cheeseburger, smothered with hot peppers.

There is so much more to this part of the birth story, but the most important part happened next, when I finally listened to my mommy gut, despite all of the false alarms and familial distractions.

My husband and I had gotten home and into our bed, and my mind started to churn in overdrive. The baby was still quiet. Something was going on. I decided that I had to call the emergency on-call doctor's line yet again, with my tail between my legs and a baby nestled in my uterus, for whom I cared and worried deeply.

I told the on-call doctor that the baby was quieter. She told me reassuringly that she was "probably fine," but if I was really worried, I could come in. I detected the slightest hint of annoyance in her voice, as I was bothering her at nine on a Saturday night. I felt guilty, but I rationalized that it was better safe than sorry and gathered up our stuff, once again, to go in for a quick check in labor and delivery.

By this point, we were old pros and figured that they would most likely send me home in an hour, so we didn't even bother bringing the dogs to my parents' or picking up my mom to join us. I was sure that I'd be home to watch my *Grey's Anatomy* rerun at eleven. With a closed cervix, thick cervix.

It's funny and kind of amazing to me; I had waited all day, toting around a stomach that contained a pit and a quiet baby, not calling the doctor, feeling like I could give it time, but as soon as I made the decision to go in and be checked, I felt a sense of urgency like I had never experienced in my life. I needed to get to the hospital as quickly as possible.

As soon as I checked in on the maternity floor, I walked as fast as I could to a delivery room, stripped off my clothes in exchange for a thin hospital gown, and rushed to the bed, so that they could hook up the fetal heart monitor, so that I could be finally soothed by the sacred sound of my daughter's heartbeat.

As soon as I heard the steady sound of her beating heart, I was able to exhale. She was OK.

A resident came in to examine me (fortunately, it was a different resident from the "head-shaker" from the night before) and did another internal pelvic exam. The exam showed that I was one centimeter dilated and 50 percent effaced. At that point, I had to laugh. I had just experienced three days of steady, solid contractions, and my cervix and uterus seemed to be giving each other the silent treatment. There was, evidently, no communication between the two whatsoever.

From the start, however, this visit to labor and delivery was different. They questioned me about the baby's movements, and, at one point, the nurse came in to give me cranberry juice, in an effort to try to encourage the baby to move. I felt drained, I felt uneasy, and then I felt water. It was the same exact water flow feeling that I had felt the evening before. I wasn't even going to mention it because of how they had dismissed me at my previous visit, the doctor saying that it was nothing, but I decided that since I was there and hooked up, I might as well tell someone that I was lying in a wet bed.

They went through the same protocol as the night before, did some tests, and went to analyze things and to speak privately as I played around on my phone, essentially waiting for the resident to come back in to tell me that I could leave.

When the door opened a few minutes later, I saw the nurse dragging in an IV pole. "I hope you're comfortable," she began. "Because you're staying. Your water broke."

"What?" I asked her, incredulous—in shock. "Are you serious? Are you sure? Like, 100 percent sure?" I think I asked her those questions eleven times each.

It was exactly what had happened the night before. I now know that my water had clearly ruptured, and they had clearly missed it.

The kind nurse told me she was serious, she was sure, and I was staying. I would be having my baby within the next twenty-four hours. I could not believe that it was finally happening. My water was broken, my contractions were steady and intensifying, my IV was in my forearm, and it was, actually, really, truly, no-doubt-about-it happening.

Yet, still, there were a few things that weren't adding up. First, the nurse was giving me another round of sugar water, this time through my IV, just so that they could try to see the baby "wake up" a bit. It was not that she wasn't moving, or that her heart wasn't beating at an ideal rate, but she wasn't having the accelerations that they liked to observe. She was fine, they assured me, but they just wanted to keep a close eye on her.

Obviously, this freaked me out, completely. I kept my eyes glued to that heart monitor, willing the numbers to rise and fall, my own heart racing as I stared. I prayed.

And then there was the whole business of my cervix. My cervix, willful and obstinate, decided to hold strong at one centimeter dilated and 50 percent effaced, which seemed comically impossible to me, considering the strength of my contractions, the duration of my labor, and the fact that my water had broken. Finally, two key people arrived: the on-call OBGYN and my mom.

The pleasant doctor introduced herself to me and told me that the baby kept moving away from the external fetal heart monitor, so they would have to attach one internally, on the baby's head.

As an aside, I should mention that my own OBGYN, a doctor who happens to be a solo practitioner, boasting a stellar record of delivering more than 90 percent of his own patients—you know, the only doctor I saw throughout my entire pregnancy—yes, the same doctor whom I saw the previous days in labor and delivery—the one who told me that he would see me, to deliver my baby, over the weekend—was not on call that evening. I had to go into battle without my trusted, white(-coated) knight. The idea of an internal fetal heart monitor scared me, as did anything that had to do with my baby's beating heart.

"Are you worried?" I asked her, eyes brimming with tears.

"I am not too too worried, but I will say that I wouldn't have gotten out of bed on a Saturday night if I were completely comfortable with this situation. I want to wake this baby up."

The doctor reached into me, stretching her hand as far as she could in order to try to place the electrode on the baby's head, and after poking around, her elbow deep inside of my body, she stopped, seemingly puzzled. She sat down on the edge of the hospital bed next to me, looked at me in the eyes, and explained that the baby was still so far up inside of me that she could not even reach the top of her head. Before I could process this information, she tried again, reaching her gloved hand into places where no one before her had ever gone. And the flood gates opened.

No, I am not talking about tears, though those were there, too. But in this case, I am referring to my water breaking, yet again. Except, this time, it was exactly the way that they show it in the movies. A huge burst of water spilled out from inside of me, soaking us and my bed.

What I did not see at that time was that there was meconium in the water, which meant, in laymen's terms, that the baby had pooped in the womb. A sign of some sort of fetal distress.

The doctor did not mention her discovery at that time, but I saw it for myself as I trekked over to the bathroom, water pouring out of me, leaving a trail of brownish water in my wake.

They changed my sopping sheets, I got back into bed, and the doctor, nurse, and I reconvened for a powwow. The doctor told me that because of my ruptured membranes and the baby's signs of distress, we needed to find a way to get the baby to come, and it did not look like my labor was progressing on its own.

Though it was hard news to hear, I did not need for her to tell me that. I was the one stuck at one centimeter dilated and 50 percent effaced for three days, despite my constant contractions.

The doctor mentioned the option of labor induction, which meant that they would give me topical medicine to soften my cervix and intravenous Pitocin in an effort to cause even stronger contractions. If all went according to plan, using this method, I would begin to dilate and efface overnight and would hopefully be in active labor by the next day.

This is the part of my story where all of those feelings kicked in. This is when something came over me; I do not know what, and I do not know how, but in that moment I knew what I had to do, and that thing had nothing to do with my hypno-birth training and a Pitocin drip.

"I need a C-section, and I need it now."

I was calm and adamant. I had been anti-intervention, in theory. But my body was not working, my baby was not thriving, and we needed to act.

The doctor and the nurse exchanged a glance. The doctor looked back and forth between my mother, my husband, and myself, and then she nodded.

"I think you're right."

The nurse took my hand as she told me, "I've never seen a first-time mom make such a smart decision in all of my years here working as a nurse. You have the right intuition."

It was at that point that they told me more about the meconium and lack of accelerations and what that could mean. It was at that point that I told them to hurry. The next thing I knew, and I mean this sincerely, my husband was dressed head to toe in sterile gear, and my dad was in the room, giving me a hug. Now, I do not know how he managed to get there so quickly; perhaps it was some kind of dad radar. And I do not know how he was allowed back into the delivery room, where you are solely permitted to have two family members; perhaps it was some kind of dad charm. But I do know that my typically swarthy-faced father was a sickening shade of off-white. He looked at me, a phony smile plastered on his pallid face, and it was at that point that I said, "OK, I guess I'm going to die."

Maybe I was being overdramatic, but after three days of labor, three sleepless nights, a horrific family accident, a seemingly endless day of a quiet baby, the funky heart monitor strip, the meconium, my drug allergies, and my paralyzing anxiety, I was convinced that I was toast.

They shuttled me into the operating room. The hospital hallway was shrouded in an eerie light, as the OBGYN, a resident, a medical student, an anesthesiologist, and my nurse wheeled me down the hall and through the big, ominous double doors. I remember seeing nurses stationed in the hallway as I was being wheeled by, and I asked them if I was going to die. They told me that I was not. I did not believe them.

As they transferred me onto the operating table, I began to shake. My husband was not with me at this time, as he was not allowed to be in the room as I got the spinal block needed for surgery, so my nurse held my hand in his place.

I later learned that for my husband, those fifteen minutes were the worst that he had experienced in his life, as he paced the halls like a madman, terrified for his wife and unborn baby, both of whom braced behind those heavy double doors.

I cannot say that I can remember the moment that my husband was allowed back with me, but I do remember telling him that I couldn't feel anything below my shoulders and that I was terribly scared. And I remember that I was shaking. And that I was nauseous. Also, I couldn't breathe. Breathing is something that we often take for granted. It is something we do, without thinking, until we cannot. And when we cannot, there are few things more horrifying—like having an unborn, but almost born, baby in distress.

Not only was my chest completely numb, making taking a deep breath nearly impossible, but the medicine that they used in the spinal block also made my nose stuff up so much that I couldn't inhale at all. My mouth became so dry that I could scarcely speak.

The anesthesiologist provided me with heavenly nectar in the form of a wet sponge, as he soaked my trembling lips, helping to ease the terrible dryness. I do not think that I had ever been more uncomfortable in my entire life. And then, before I knew it, the anesthesiologist was instructing my husband to take out the camera and to hold it over the curtain that separated my head from my abdomen. It was time. The anesthesiologist told me that my baby would be delivered in a matter of minutes. I was so terrified that I could not even speak, and I could barely stop shaking enough to nod my head.

And then the entire world changed.

I heard my daughter's voice. Her cry was fast and staccato, and more beautiful than any music that I had ever heard. She sounded so strong, her voice already so powerful, and I knew that she was OK. At that point, the OBGYN told me that her cord had been wrapped around her neck two times. We were very lucky that we had gotten her out when we did.

I wish that I could say that it was at that moment that I forgot all of my discomfort, instead simply staring into my daughter's gorgeous blue eyes as I told my husband how much I loved and cherished him. That did happen, but much later. At this point, my shaking got so bad that I couldn't form words, and my nausea had turned into relentless heaving.

All I kept saying to my husband was that I was so sorry I could not enjoy the experience with him—with them; I was so sorry that I felt so ill. All that he kept saying was "She's so beautiful. She's so beautiful." And he cried. He cried enough for both of us. And he loved her. He loved her enough for both of us. He didn't have to, for I loved her insanely already—I just couldn't express it yet. I was still on the table, broken, needing to be put back together.

At one point, which felt like it was several hours later, I asked the doctor, who was still out of my view, behind the blue curtain, if she could give me something to help me with my nausea.

"Oh, don't worry," she said. "You'll feel much better once I put your uterus back in."

Back in? I hadn't been aware that it was out. But she did, and the nausea abated, and I was sewn and stapled and, finally, wheeled back out of the operating room and into the delivery room, where it had all began.

And the rest, as they say, was the start to my happily ever after.

In the delivery room I saw my husband; my parents; my sister, who had rushed to the hospital from her college apartment downtown; and my Mom Mom, who came running, in the middle of the night, to be by my side, as only Mom Moms can do. We all hugged, and cried, and they showed me pictures of my daughter, as I hadn't been able to take in her beautiful face while I was still on the operating table. Another thing that I did not know at that time was that when my husband went out to greet my family after the baby was born, he walked down the hall crying. When my family saw him, they were sick with worry. They did not realize that he was sobbing tears of joy until he held them and said, "She's so beautiful."

And she is.

"Annabelle Lily Starr says hello," he said, and though I was not there to see his face, I can only imagine how brightly he was shining from the inside out. From the moment she was born, our Belle was the most amazingly beautiful, angelic, perfect baby that there ever was. My daughter was born on April 18, 2010, at 2:22 in the morning. She weighed seven pounds, twelve ounces and was twenty-one inches long.

She came into the world with brown hair; big, shining eyes; a heart-shaped face; and lips like Cupid's arrow. She has the sweetest, most edible chin imaginable. And despite the fact that I just extolled her virtues, I have to admit that we look strikingly similar.

Belle radiates goodness and lights up the universe. She was welcomed into the world by our parents, grandparents, siblings, and friends, and those loved ones who are no longer with us, like the one for whom she is named—the name that we chose for her, so many years before, while sitting on the beach, as the sun was setting.

Annabelle.

And then there were three.

Part II
A HARD STORY

2

❖ ❖

Professional Perspective
on Prenatal Distress

WHAT IS PRENATAL DISTRESS?

Dr. Amy Wenzel, an expert in the field of perinatal distress and editor of *The Oxford Handbook of Perinatal Psychology*, provided me with an incredible amount of insight and information as the collaborator for parts of this book. Dr. Wenzel is a psychologist with a thriving practice, an accomplished author, and a mother, who shares the desire to help others so that they can be set up for success. I consulted with Dr. Wenzel in order to write this book. She gave me both clinical research information and examples of her own experiences with patients, in order to best illustrate these perinatal afflictions. In this chapter (and others) I will be using her insight and sharing information from her books, with her express permission, as I paraphrase some of her written words, as well as the words from our conversations together and tape-recorded interviews. Dr. Wenzel and I met in her clinical office and spoke over the phone many times from 2015 to 2017 in our quest to provide robust data, share information, and gather as many salient suggestions as possible. It is because of Dr. Wenzel's contributions that this book offers actionable advice, rather than solely one woman's story.

According to Dr. Wenzel, depression affects approximately 9–13 percent of pregnant women. Additionally, pregnant women can suffer from anxiety, panic attacks, obsessions and compulsions, post-traumatic stress disorder, and other psychopathological disorders.

In pregnancy women experience changes of every kind: physical, psychological, behavioral, and more. Every pregnancy affects a woman differently, but there are some commonalities that studies have shown to be correlated with the prenatal period. In *The Oxford Handbook of Perinatal Psychology*, Dr. Wenzel discusses these profound perinatal changes. She explains that during the prenatal period, psychological and physical symptoms can be mutually influential.

First, there are the mood changes that women experience during pregnancy. As Dr. Wenzel has explained, "There is no set of discrete, universal stages for psychological adaptation to pregnancy. Nevertheless, research has identified certain psychological tasks that are typically encountered during pregnancy and the transition to motherhood." Women must reconcile the boundaries between their own bodies and their growing babies, which can be a very difficult adjustment. In so many ways, they are one, but, in truth, a pregnant woman is a vessel for another life. As fundamental as it may sound, the first psychological step to occur when a woman becomes pregnant is her actual recognition of the pregnancy. Dr. Wenzel's research shows that, according to the Pregnancy Risk Assessment Monitoring System (PRAMS), more than 90 percent of women do recognize that they are pregnant within the first twelve weeks.

Another prominent prenatal psychological change involves body image. As a woman's body morphs and grows to accommodate her growing fetus, she must get used to looking and feeling different from what was normal prior to becoming pregnant. In some cases, as Dr. Wenzel has explained, a woman will feel positive about the changes in her body's shape. For such a woman, the bodily changes indicate that she is doing something good: growing a healthy baby inside of her. In some cases, she will feel a sense of accomplishment, prompting a feeling of achievement in herself and her body's changes. Conversely, other women have negative reactions to the changes in their shapes and sizes. For example, a woman may not feel like herself and therefore struggle with her identity. Women who experience negative body image issues during their pregnancies usually fear excessive weight gain, feel less sexually attractive, and struggle with how they identify, physically, as a woman.

Additionally, there are the somatic changes that a woman experiences. Some common pregnancy symptoms are nausea, vomiting, and fatigue. A woman may also be more sensitive to smells, which prompt the other aforementioned symptoms. According to one study, 70–85 percent of pregnant women experience nausea, or what is commonly referred to as "morning sickness," and 50 percent of women vomit as a result of their pregnancy.[1]

Needless to say, being pregnant changes many things in a woman's life, which can make coping difficult. Along with the psychological changes that a woman may experience, there are inevitable biological changes that occur during pregnancy. Pregnancy symptoms can range from a nuisance level to severe, and women have little control over how the pregnancy hormones will affect them during this time.

It is important to note that "prolonged bouts of physical illness or chronic pain may adversely affect mood and may frequently lead to depression" in a pregnant woman.[2] This is to say that the worse a woman feels physically during her pregnancy, the more likely she is to develop some level of prenatal distress.

Prenatal anxiety and depression can be debilitating for women. Having a preexisting mental health condition is a commonly accepted risk factor for prenatal distress disorders, but a woman's age, hormone levels, and life circumstances all contribute to these prenatal issues.

In our conversations, Dr. Wenzel said that the peak age for a woman to experience prenatal distress is thirty years old, which falls directly during her childbearing years. Pregnancy hormones are often contributing factors or responsible for prenatal mood disorders. Research shows that the woman's brain is actually biologically affected during pregnancy. Her neurotransmitters are altered, which will impact her ability to regulate emotions, as myriad chemicals and hormones are fluctuating constantly.

Prenatal depression can be difficult to diagnose, especially for those women with a preexisting condition or a history of depression, as many of the symptoms are the same.

Anxiety is also a common form of prenatal distress. Dr. Wenzel says that 39 percent of women suffer from some sort of prenatal mood disorder. However, it can be hard to tease apart statistically normal anxiety and stress levels from diagnosable disorders, as pregnancy can be a time for increased anxiety for women without actual *clinical* prenatal anxiety disorder. With all of the psychological and hormonal changes that a woman is facing during pregnancy, some level of worry is to be expected. It is when that anxiety becomes disruptive to her life and ability to function that it should be identified, diagnosed, and treated.

RISK FACTORS

Dr. Wenzel explains that risk factors for prenatal distress are complex, as they are sometimes intuitive, yet, at other times, surprising. There is no one factor that determines whether a woman will experience prenatal distress. People who struggle with mental health problems are usually characterized by factors that make them vulnerable to experiencing emotional distress, and emotional distress is realized in the context of life stress. Pregnancy is a stressful life event for most women, and a scare, like bleeding during pregnancy, can certainly propel those vulnerabilities into a mental health problem.

The most significant risk factor for prenatal distress is a woman's history of anxiety, depression, or other mental health problems. For many women, prenatal distress is actually a continuation of a mental health condition, one from which they had been suffering prior to pregnancy. This is the most common manifestation of prenatal distress. Moreover, if a woman has experienced perinatal issues in the past (with prenatal distress, postpartum depression, or both), then she has a much higher risk for a recurrence during a subsequent pregnancy.

An interesting risk factor for prenatal distress is the degree to which a woman experiences mood reactivity associated with her menstrual cycle. Extensive research has aimed to identify various hormone levels that are associated with perinatal distress, and, interestingly, data has been inconclusive. In actuality, it seems that there is no one hormone level that is directly associated with perinatal distress; rather, certain woman are more sensitive to rapid changes in their hormone levels. If a woman experiences substantial mood reactivity related to her cycles, then she is at a greater risk of developing prenatal distress.

In addition to a woman's history of mental health problems in general, as well as perinatal mental health problems specifically, it is important to consider psychological risk factors. These risk factors include personality styles, ways of viewing oneself and the world, and ways of approaching problems that can be more or less helpful when one is faced with stress, life challenges, and adversity. An example of a psychological risk factor is the intolerance of uncertainty. Although most people experience some anxiety when they are faced with uncertainty, people who are characterized by the intolerance of uncertainty experience significant anxious apprehension, worry, and catastrophic thinking when dealing with the unknown. It is not difficult to see how women who struggle with an intolerance of uncertainty would experience a tremendous amount of anxiety during pregnancy, to the extent that they experience little joy associated with pregnancy milestones for fear that something will soon go wrong.

WARNING SIGNS

Dr. Wenzel explained to me that a warning sign is an indicator that a person is experiencing emotional distress at a level that would be diagnosed as having a mental health problem. The inability to fulfill one or more life responsibilities is a warning sign for an array of mental health problems, including prenatal distress. However, it is not a dysfunction when a woman is experiencing pregnancy-related exhaustion or variable mood shift from hormonal changes. A sign of true suffering is when things are obviously starting to slip in a woman's life, whether at work, in her home life, or, if applicable, with her other children.

It is important to note that every woman experiences anxiety during pregnancy. A moderate level of anxiety is actually the norm during this sensitive period in a woman's life. However, it is a sign of prenatal distress when a woman's anxiety is causing interference in her life. For example, when a woman seems anxious all the time, is in need of a great deal of reassurance, or is having difficulty completing her usual responsibilities due to associated symptoms of anxiety (e.g., concentration difficulties), then she may be experiencing prenatal distress. If her intrusive thoughts are pushing out her necessary thoughts, for example, then she could potentially end up being neglectful of her prenatal care, visits to the OBGYN, and other health measures that are encouraged for a healthy pregnancy.

As previously stated, physiologically and psychologically, every pregnant woman is going through a great deal of changes, so it is to be expected that there will be times of anxious apprehension, exhaustion, or sadness. It is when the distress persists or worsens that there is an indication of a true problem.

TREATMENT

Women who experience prenatal distress are encouraged to seek help from their support system, from a professional, or, ideally, from both. A holistic approach, involving as many members of a support team as is indicated (or possible), would be ideal.

First, on the personal side, a support system is a very important treatment tool for women suffering from any form of perinatal distress. For the partner or family member of an anxious or depressed pregnant woman, the best suggestion is to lead with compassion. Be gentle. Collaborate with her, rather than simply tell her to get help. Perceiving oneself as inadequate is one of the worst things that a pregnant woman can experience, so let her know that her emotional experiences are understandable and that there are resources to help.

Clinically, there are myriad treatment approaches. Dr. Wenzel specializes in cognitive behavioral therapy, but she also uses techniques from dialectical behavior therapy, trauma treatment, and psychotherapy.

For some women, traditional talk therapy is not enough, and they must take medication in order to stabilize their moods during pregnancy. For many women, this can be upsetting, as they do not want to put anything foreign or chemical into their bodies while they are pregnant. In some cases, a woman has to decide whether to stay on her anxiety or depression medication during her pregnancy, or whether she can find other ways to cope without it. In other cases, women without preexisting mental health conditions may be encouraged to start taking medication in an effort to regulate their emotions.

Because of this conflict, one that is both internal and external, psychological and medical, the American Psychiatric Association and the American College of Obstetricians and Gynecologists teamed up to write a comprehensive report on the use of medication—specifically antidepressants—during pregnancy. Their goal was "to address the maternal and neonatal risks of both depression and antidepressant exposure and develop algorithms for periconceptional and antenatal management."[3] As their article states:

> Both depression symptoms and the use of antidepressant medications during pregnancy have been associated with negative consequences for the newborn. Infants born to women with depression have increased risk for irritability, less activity and attentiveness, and fewer facial expressions compared with those born to mothers without depression. Depression and its symptoms are also associated with fetal growth change and shorter gestation periods. And while available research still leaves some questions unanswered, some studies have linked fetal malformations, cardiac defects, pulmonary hypertension, and reduced birth weight to antidepressant use during pregnancy.[4]

The article also states that approximately 13 percent of pregnant women have reported taking an antidepressant at some point during their pregnancy.[5]

The article goes on to say:

Ob-gyns are the front-line physicians for most pregnant women and may be the first to make a diagnosis of depression or to observe depressive symptoms getting worse. In the past, reproductive health practitioners have felt ill equipped to treat these patients because of the lack of available guidance concerning the management of depressed women during pregnancy. . . . This joint report bridges the gap by summarizing current research on various depression treatment methods and can assist clinicians in decision-making. Many people—physicians and women alike—will be glad to know that their choices go beyond "medication or nothing."[6]

Prenatal anxiety can be a great predictor of postpartum depression.[7] This is according to a study that was aimed at predicting whether the presence of prenatal anxiety was a significant predictor of distress post-birth, using the Brief Measure of Worry Severity (BMWS), which is a brief and valid self-report measure used to assess severe and dysfunctional worry.[8] Furthermore, this measurement is obtained when participants complete and self-report, and then clinicians rate measures of anxiety and diagnostic interviews for generalized anxiety disorder (GAD).[9]

In fact, the study examining the relationship between prenatal and postnatal mood disorders found a rather stunning correlation: by taking a sample of 748 women and analyzing them during their third trimesters of pregnancy and again at eight weeks postpartum, the researchers determined that "women with high antenatal anxiety on the BMWS were 2.6 times more likely" to have postpartum depression than the women who had lower levels of anxiety during their pregnancies.[10]

Echoing the earlier insight from the American Psychiatric Association and the American College of Obstetricians and Gynecologists, Christine Dunkel Schetter and Lynlee Tanner point to severe risk factors for both mother and child, stemming from anxiety, depression, and stress during pregnancy: "Anxiety in pregnancy is associated with shorter gestation and has adverse implications for fetal neurodevelopment and child outcomes."[11]

In summary, scientists—medical and psychological—have found that the less anxious and distressed a woman is during her pregnancy, the better the outcome will be for her and her baby. With risk factors for both physical and mental health conditions for the mother as well as the fetus, it is important to manage a woman's prenatal distress appropriately. Ideally, this can be done through proper identification, support, and therapy. In other, more severe cases, pregnant women can take antidepressant medications prescribed by their physicians, when it is indicated that the risk of depression outweighs any possible risk to the growing baby. It is a balancing act, but with continued research, increased awareness, a commitment to compassionate healthcare, and additional comprehensive studies on maternal, fetal, and pediatric health, women can be set up for and guided through successful prenatal and postpartum periods.

3

❖ ❖

Uncomfortably Numb

The Beginning of My Prenatal Distress

Prenatal distress refers to anxiety or depression during pregnancy that reaches a point at which it causes life interference or substantial personal distress. I did not know that such conditions existed until they swallowed me whole.

"House, then baby, then dog." That was my refrain. My husband wanted all of those things; I was sure about one, less so about the others.

In December 2012 we bought the house that we had always wanted; it was in that magical neighborhood where Kenny and I had grown up, around the corner from where my parents live. It has charming, unique features like French doors and pegboard wood floors and molding, and, best of all, we could afford it because most buyers could not see past the horrible peach paint and scratched linoleum floors. I poured my heart into refurbishing and redecorating this house. On a limited budget, we were able to make substantial changes, both structural (central air!) and aesthetic (every surface painted!), and we finally moved into our new home in the first month of 2013.

At the time of our move, Annabelle was two and a half years old. In some ways, she and I had created our own enchanted world, filled with tutus and dance parties and sparkly shoes. She was my Belle, in every sense of the word. She was an incredible little girl; she started talking at six months old, could identify a song by its first chord, and had an empathy and wisdom that belied her young age and small stature.

Belle and I were more than mother and daughter; we were a team. We were fiercely bonded. I breastfed her for eighteen months, which, in my mind, was a testament to our connection. All of the anxiety during my pregnancy with her had been more than worth it, as she was the living embodiment of my lifelong dreams. I reassured myself about said anxiety, attributing my hypervigilance to her awesomeness; I think that somewhere, deep inside my brain, I thought that if I had, in fact, had deli meat or champagne during those nine months, perhaps Belle would have been different in some way. I am going to go out on a limb in saying that now, in hindsight, I will give that notion a big "no."

I was always protective of Belle, and it pained me when she felt scared, sad, or sick. But as she grew from newborn to infant to baby to toddler to little kid, I also grew. I became increasingly confident and competent, called the doctor less, and trusted my own intuition more. We had a nice rhythm, and though Kenny was always an incredibly devoted, loving father, Belle and I had our own thing going. I was hers as much as she was mine.

As soon as we moved and settled into our new dream home, things changed. It was at this time that Kenny's desire for another baby amped up a few notches. He was not only ready but also eager. While I had been the one leading the charge to get pregnant with Belle, he started to push for a second baby and felt that with our little girl verging on three years old, it was the right time for us to "start trying."

In addition to Kenny's encouragement, I noticed that all of my mom peers were either pregnant with or raising their second children. All of the other kids in Belle's preschool class were becoming big brothers and big sisters, and it seemed as though each week one of her friends would bring in a photo of their new sibling. Feeling guilty about this, I sent Belle in to school with a photograph of her new bedroom. She got a lot of attention for her very cool, chic kilim-style rug from Pottery Barn Teen, and her kind teachers hung up her photo on the wall, right next to the collection of baby photos. I wanted my daughter to have something about which to feel special and proud—I just did not necessarily want to have to grow that "something" in my uterus at that time.

It was not as though I did not want to expand our family. I love children. I dreamed of what it would be like for Belle to have a sibling, and I thought of her as the ideal candidate for big sisterhood. My hesitancy was deeper than that. My brutal truth is this: I was terrified. I was scared about having another nine months of anxiety, worrying about whether the baby would be safe or if, like my daughter, he would have the cord wrapped around his neck twice, causing him to stop moving on the day of delivery. I was petrified of a repeat cesarean section; yet that was my only option. I was not going to be a candidate for a vaginal birth after cesarean (VBAC), and so I had to gear up for another major surgery. I hated my daughter's birth; I couldn't breathe, as my spinal was placed too high, numbing my chest, and I was unable to hold her for hours, not allowing me to experience those coveted first moments of bonding and breastfeeding. I was very anxious about how our triangle would morph into a square. Basically, there were not many things that I was not nervous about, except for getting pregnant. Unlike the first time, I was not worried, as I was in no rush and on no timeline.

So, of course, we got pregnant the first month that we tried. To be more candid, it was a one-shot deal. After the experience of trying to conceive my daughter, I knew what signs to look for, and so when I recognized that I was in my "fertile window," I sent my husband a text at work: "I think I am ovulating, FYI."

It was an incredibly romantic seduction.

I knew that I was pregnant almost instantly, even when an early test had a negative result. When I took that test and saw only one line appear, I felt a pang of displaced disappointment but was not convinced. I kept myself distracted, which was easy with a two-year-old.

I had a strange intuition—mommy gut, as they say—but I also had noticed a different sort of strange gut change that happened right away: my normally cavernous belly button was not as deep. I first assumed that I had, perhaps, gained some weight. But in the back of my mind I was aware that the only other time that my belly button had morphed similarly was during my first pregnancy. It's a uterus thing.

Despite my negative pregnancy test, I *felt* pregnant, with swollen, tender breasts and excessive tiredness. I can remember sitting at my kitchen table with my mom as she tried to assuage my disappointment about "failing" during our first month of trying.

"These things don't happen right away," she said.

"But, Mom," I began to explain, "I really think I am pregnant. I know that the test said that I am not, but I just have this feeling." And it was at this time that I really started to *want* it. My apathy and trepidation were waning as my excitement was brewing.

I decided to retest a week after my period was late, on a cold March morning, when I was home alone with Belle. I peed on the home pregnancy test stick and saw a dark line appear on the right side of the test window. I was confused, at first.

"Isn't the control line on the left?" I asked myself.

As I stared, perplexed, at my test, a second line—the actual control line—began to appear, slightly fainter than the first. And then it hit me. Two clear lines. It was positive. I was pregnant. I was so pregnant that the HCG levels could not even wait for the control to inform me.

"I'm pregnant," I said, breathlessly, while standing, pants down, in my bathroom.

"I'm Cinderella," my wide-eyed little girl replied.

I touched my belly. It was no longer just a body part but the vessel for Belle's sibling. It was magical. All of my doubt washed away, leaving room for excitement and dreams.

Kenny had been out at an elaborate brunch, and so when he returned home, we had the opportunity to surprise him. I had Belle present him with a wrapped box. He opened it cavalierly, expecting to find a project made from a Popsicle stick, not a pee stick. When he pulled out the test, he said, "What?" in the way that sounds like a question but really is an answer.

We looked at each other.

This was getting real.

We were able to tell our family members in much more exciting ways the second time around than we had with my daughter. First, we video chatted with my sister in New York. We waved the pregnancy test in front of my small iPhone screen, and she jumped up and down. She had been in the "it's time to have another baby and I can't wait for you to do it" camp for several months, and so this was a dream come true for her as well. We asked my dad to come over to "look at our new sconces" while I secretly perched the pregnancy test on the mantel. He hugged me tightly, and then more gently, and told me that I looked thin and to make sure that I was eating enough (so much for my belly button theory). We called my mom, who had just landed in St. Thomas for a trip with her parents.

"I knew it!" she said.

It was really exciting. I was really excited. It was as if, almost instantly, my fears dissipated into a soothing, brilliant warmth that enveloped all of me. I felt like this amazing new stage was beginning, and I was over-whelmed with a feeling of love toward my poppy seed–sized embryo from the start, as I was aware, then, of the power of a mother's love. I thought that it was another girl.

But as the first week went on, my excitement slowly morphed into anxiety. It was not nervousness about having another baby but the anxiety that something bad would happen.

"I just want to know that everything is going to be OK."

The first time that I really felt affected by the anxiety was during the following week while at work. A young child ran to me for a big hug and, in doing so, inadvertently knocked into my stomach. I remember panicking. Despite all that I know intellectually about a baby's safety inside the amniotic sack, I freaked out that he had harmed my little growing embryo. Despite constant reassurance from my husband, I could not shake the anxiety. I believe that that is what sets this anxiety apart from the fears and worries and doubts that I experienced during my pregnancy with Belle: Once an anxious thought came into my mind, I was unable to let it go. I would ruminate, going over and over the painful or scary subject in my head, unable to stop the intrusive thoughts from creeping in. My anxiety even served to distract me; I could not get out of my own mind.

I remember being so comforted by my uncomfortable pregnancy symptoms. How is that for an oxymoron? Morning sickness, to me, meant that there was a growing baby inside of me with HCG levels rising. So, when I woke up feeling less nauseated than I had been the day before, I started to get the panicky feeling once again. The cycle of rumination began anew, and I worried that perhaps my levels were dropping and that something was not right with my baby.

I called my OBGYN's office and spoke to the nurse practitioner.

I explained my symptoms to her, or lack thereof, and told her that I would like to be seen in the office for an ultrasound and bloodwork, just to confirm my pregnancy and that the levels were rising appropriately. I told her that this would give me comfort, hoping for some compassionate care, but instead she told me that I was "probably fine" and to "keep an eye out for blood." Blood would be bad. My request for an ultrasound was denied. This did not provide comfort; instead, it made me even more scared.

Though I kept a lot of my fearful feelings inside, I finally confided in a trusted fellow mom friend. I will be honest—this was not planned or a strategic move aimed at self-care; rather, once my hardened exterior cracked the slightest amount, it all came pouring out like a deluge. When I was five and a half weeks pregnant, I went to my standing sushi date with my aforementioned close friend and two other women, who are also moms. This was a monthly ritual for us, and something that I typically looked forward to very much. However, I was so lost in my own head that I might as well have been a million miles away, unable to concentrate on creative Maki rolls and preschool gossip. Though I tried to mask it, I had been uncharacteristically quiet throughout the dinner. Though my one close friend knew that I was pregnant—something that I could not hide from her, considering the nature of our relationship—I had not shared the news with my other dining companions. Regardless, it was clear that something was amiss. I was off. I was so wrapped up in my intrusive thoughts that I could not focus at all and asked to leave a bit early, blaming my fatigue on long work hours. This was a terrible excuse, as at the time I was teaching preschool, but I needed a change of scenery, as my sunken sushi table was beginning to feel like a subterranean suffocation device. My close friend left with me, and after some quiet small talk during our short ride home she called me out, just as I pulled into her driveway.

"What is going on? You were so far away tonight," she asked me, kindly.

I started to talk and the words got stuck in my throat, choking me from deep within.

And then, finally, I let go. I burst into tears. All of the pent-up fear came rushing out in torrents and I found my voice.

I said, "I am so scared that something is going to go wrong." My fear was completely irrational. I had no reason to believe that there was an issue, or that there would be; yet I was tangled up in worry like it was a strand of necklaces, unable to be teased apart. She could not understand my anxiety but expressed compassion nonetheless. I explained to her that I knew that I was feeling disproportionally and unfoundedly terrified. I was having a normal pregnancy with typical symptoms.

"Everything is going to be OK," she said. "And if it isn't, then it wasn't meant to be."

Her words were the kind of words that are meant to be soothing—that are said with the best of intentions—but that, in actuality, are scary as hell. I couldn't focus on her first comment, instead ruminating over the latter. I did not hear the reassurance, but rather the "if" and "then" and applied subtext there, involving every possible scary scenario that my quick moving brain could possibly conjure up. I worried that it was possible that it was not, in fact, meant to be. I worried about losing something—someone—before it could even begin.

I believe that part of my severe anxiety was that the pregnancy experience was so different from the first time around. Then I was monitored closely, as I had been seeing specialists. When I was trying to get pregnant with Belle and then finally conceived her, I saw her on an ultrasound at five, six, seven, and eight weeks. I saw the tiny grain of rice inside the black bubble that was my womb. And then, when her heart started to beat, I watched that tiny grain of rice start to flicker, at 160 beats per minute. I saw the baby when she looked like a teddy bear, with a railroad track for a spine and the tiniest of limb buds beginning to form. I saw those buds turn into arms and then hands, and I even saw her "waving," as they say. But since my second time around was a "normal" conception and pregnancy, I would have to wait until I was ten weeks to even see if there was anything in there. That, to me, was horrifying. I worried constantly. I called the OB-GYN several more times, with questions like "I feel slightly less morning sick again today, is that normal?" and "Are you *sure* that I shouldn't come in for a blood test to check my HCG levels?"

The nurse's reply was consistent: "As long as you don't see blood, you are fine."

"But I am not as nauseated. Does that mean that my levels are dropping? I am really scared. Can I just come in for a quick ultrasound?" I asked.

The nurse practitioner tried to reassure me, but her answer remained the same: I would have to wait for my ten-week appointment.

Her words kept echoing through my head. *"As long as you don't see blood, you are fine."*

Reassuring, that was not. I waited and waited and waited for blood to appear. And then, a week later, during my seventh week of pregnancy, it did. On a Sunday night in mid-March—as the sun started to set on St. Patrick's Day—there was a drop of blood on my toilet paper.

This was something that had never happened to me during my first pregnancy. I was spotting. Not a lot, but enough. The blood was not the type of blood that the nurse practitioner had told me to watch out for. It was brown and in a very small amount, but it was there.

The spotting started while I was at my parents' house. We had a family dinner with my cousins. I had walked in and told them, in confidence, our exciting news. We were eating Chinese food for dinner. I was cramping, went to use the bathroom, and I saw a little bit of blood.

Since it was a Sunday night, I had to call the emergency OBGYN service and the doctor on call told me, without a shred of compassion, "Well, either you're having a miscarriage or you're not. So you can do one of two things: You can wait until your OB's office is open tomorrow and see him then, or you can go to the ER. And if you *are* having a miscarriage, there isn't anything that we can do about it, so you can just wait until tomorrow to get checked out."

Obviously, we went to the emergency room.

St. Patrick's Day night is not a good time to find yourself needing to visit the emergency room. It was horrifying. The emergency room was so crowded that I was not even given a room; rather, I had to sit on a gurney in the hallway, under a few layers of blankets in order to keep me warm. The nurses did not understand that I was not shivering because I was cold but that the adrenaline pumping through my body was causing me to literally shake with fear.

As I sat on the hospital bed in the hallway, with my husband seated on the other end, fiddling around on his phone, I started to worry for my daughter. What would I tell her if I lost the baby?

When I asked my husband this question, I could not stop the tears from forming in my eyes and flowing down my cheeks in huge drops, like a cartoon character, albeit a very sad, shivering cartoon character having blood drawn in the hallway of an emergency room.

My husband told me not to worry. That we would "cross that bridge if we come to it" and that he was sure that everything was fine. He reminded me that spotting was normal.

After they drew my blood, they gave me a blind ultrasound, so that while a technician examined me with a transvaginal wand, she had her computer monitor facing away from me. Typically, in a healthy pregnancy, the first ultrasound is a special, magical experience. Instead, I was being probed, at my most vulnerable time, and listening to the tech as she would zoom in on certain areas of my uterus and ovaries, take a screen shot of the area and move the wand around mercilessly inside of me. I closed my eyes and imagined a flickering grain of rice before her, willing it to be there—willing life to be inside of me.

As the nurse continued to move her magic wand around, snapping picture after picture of the unknown, I looked up at her and pleaded.

"Is the baby OK?" I asked through tears.

"I am sorry, but I cannot give you any information. You will have to wait to speak with your doctor after he gets the report from the radiologist."

"Can you just give me a wink?" I asked. She did not.

Naturally, I assumed the worst. I know that there are strict guidelines about what a technician is and is not allowed to say, but I would have appreciated a blanket "Everything is going to be OK, so don't worry!" to assuage my mounting fears. She wheeled me out of her small, dark room without another word.

I had more rounds of bloodwork and internal exams, and finally, hours later, the emergency room attending physician came into our room.

"Well, the good news is that your levels are all normal. The heart rate is 123, which is perfectly fine for this stage in pregnancy and—" I cut him off.

"Wait. So there is a heartbeat? The baby is OK?" I asked, incredulously.

"Yes. The baby looks good. It looks like a little Cheerio right now, but there is a heartbeat and the sac has formed and all of your levels are great."

"Can I see?" I asked him, choking on my tears.

"I can't print out the ultrasound picture like they do in the OB's office," he explained. "But if you want to come see the photos on my computer screen, you can do that."

And so, unlike any other experience I had had previously, I first saw my baby, standing in the crowded nurse's station of an even more crowded emergency room, peering over the shoulder of the doctor as he pulled up an image on his low-resolution computer screen. I remember seeing a black background and, like he said, a small round circle, resembling a Cheerio.

"That's our baby," I said.

But something was still wrong. Despite all of the tests and reassurances and the fact that we confirmed that my baby was in my uterus, with a beating heart and growing appropriately, I did not feel the elation or relief that I was expecting. It had been an incredibly intense, scary episode for me. I was still reeling. And, at the same time, I have never felt more alone.

And after that night, I went numb.

4

❖ ❖

"I Didn't Know Exactly What It Was, But I Knew to Fear It"

My Prenatal Anxiety and Depression

After my traumatic emergency room visit for spotting during pregnancy—called a "possible miscarriage" on the paperwork with which I was sent home from the hospital—I went from a state of high anxiety to complete numbness with regard to my baby.

It is very hard for me to write this; in fact, it is agonizing and feels like a betrayal. But the truth is that this trauma changed things for me. It caused me to completely detach from the baby inside of me. Clearly it was a defense mechanism. I knew intellectually that spotting is a very normal occurrence in many healthy pregnancies, but this threw (the already very anxious) me overboard.

Instead of caring more, I cared less. This was not a conscious thing, mind you; it is only something I can recognize in hindsight. But I stopped feeling for the baby. Everything in my life just stopped. I was swimming through my days, suffocating under water, drowning a slow proverbial death. I was so oxygen deprived that my sensations dulled to nothingness.

Except I did feel severe morning sickness. To put things into context, I was hesitant to take so much as an acetaminophen (a drug deemed safe) during my first pregnancy; yet, during my second, I had to take prescription antinausea medication around the clock in order to keep my vomiting down to ten times a day. I was crumbling from the inside out.

The numbness and discomfort only intensified at twelve weeks, when the perinatal ultrasound tech told me that he saw "something between the legs." By "something," he meant a penis.

Twelve weeks is very early to find out a baby's sex (that typically happens at the twenty-week anatomy scan). I was in shock. Not only was I having another baby, not only was I puking all day, every day, not only was I feeling very mixed emotions, if anything at all, but a boy? I had come from such a girl family. We quoted *Dirty Dancing* regularly, wore tutus, and had only a hot pink high chair. I couldn't believe it. Nothing was going as planned. And that feeling of incredulity continued.

A symptom of this agony was that I stopped being protective of my growing baby. Let me be clear that I was certainly responsible in my pregnancy, avoiding deli meat, alcohol, and heavy lifting, but I was not nearly as cautious or loving as I had been to my first child. I didn't sing to my belly every night. I didn't read the baby stories. I did not paint canvases for him with words of love. I did not hum his name through my head all day with glee. I did not call the OBGYN or nearly crash Google with crazy questions. And though I loved feeling my son kick and move (his transverse position allowed me to feel everything), I felt that the sensation was "cool" as opposed to "exciting" or "reassuring."

I was not sure that I could love another child. I was not sure that I could love a boy.

As time went on, I sank further into a deep ocean of pain and uncertainty. I still could not breathe but learned to accommodate the feeling, as if I were sucking air through a tiny straw. My lungs burned; my heart ached.

To some people, I made light of the situation, trying to make jokes with my teeth gritted into a smile: "I don't know what I am going to do with a boy! I hope he likes to play dress-up!" Or "Oh no, I'm not pregnant; I am just smuggling a basketball," which was more of a testament to how I looked. I was described as a bowling ball with sticks coming out.

To a few others, I confided my secret: I really wasn't sure that I wanted him.

When my mom and I went shopping for the baby's layette, we went to a nice department store, an experience that should have been fun and exciting. It was where we had bought our entire, beloved baby wardrobe for Belle, and yet the sentimentality was lost on me, replaced with disdain and resentment.

I was angry that the baby boy clothing seemed to me like it was so much less cute than the baby girl clothing. Everything was light blue or had a teddy bear on it, and I decided that I hated light blue and teddy bears. We left the department store that day without a single item for my son. I could not find one thing that I deemed acceptable, and I felt a combination of sadness and anger. Everything was going wrong. Nothing, nothing at all—not even onesies—felt right. I hated teddy bears so much.

Some of this was certainly circumstantial, but much of what was going on in me was hormonal. Oh, the hormones. The crushing hormones that managed to sneak up on me, embracing me in their anxiety-producing grasp. I was suffering from what I now know is called prenatal distress. I was so down. Not all of the time, but some of the time. A lot of the time. Most of the time. I couldn't focus on my family. I had scary thoughts. I could say that I was "OK." I could still recognize myself. But the stress was nearly blinding.

This pain manifested itself most acutely when I got my first migraine with a complex aura. The episode started on a summer afternoon during my seventh month of pregnancy. I was coloring with my daughter when dark spots started to appear in my line of sight. It was as if I had just stared into the sun but could not get my eyes to readjust. I called the doctor, who initially expressed concern that I was having a stroke. While on the phone, the darkness started to morph into flickering lights, like a shining film reel, distorting my vision, and with a vague headache creeping in, he told me that I was having a migraine and to lie down in a dark room.

Fortunately, with my parents living around the corner, my mom was able to come over within minutes so that she could simultaneously help me to care for Belle and assuage my growing sense of worry.

The three of us cuddled up in my darkened bedroom. An old movie played on the television in the background, distracting my daughter, and my mom engaged me in conversation as a means of distraction.

I started to notice a problem—I was trying to convey a specific story to her and I was losing about a word per sentence, meaning that I could not find the right way to say what I was trying to say.

This symptom worsened, and I was soon experiencing one of the scariest episodes in my entire life: I lost my ability to speak. I can imagine that anyone reading this who knows me personally will insert a joke here about me and my being horrified at the thought of not being able to talk, but this was the real deal, full loss of communication. Not only could I not speak verbally, but I also could not text message, and the notes I was sending to my husband with updates came out in gibberish. I kept trying to form sentences, and words would come out, but not the right ones—not words that made any sense. And I felt paralyzed and powerless, and when it finally started to abate I expressed how terrifying it had been. My loved ones had also been concerned. The speech loss morphed into numbness, and then the intense pain finally hit. The pain was a relief, and the best part of my migraine. The aura was far worse, and I still live in fear of having another episode.

I made an appointment to see a specialist. I saw different doctors as the pregnancy wore on (and I use that diction intentionally, because that is what it did—it wore me down). Many doctors were concerned for me after the birth, but no one took my situation as seriously as the neurologist I saw after my migraine. We sat in his office as I described my aura, and then I told him, through sobs, that I was not sure that I wanted to have a baby. I was thirty-three weeks pregnant, and I told him how terrified I was for my repeat C-section. I told him that I didn't even want a second child. I told him that something didn't feel right—that I had not felt right in months. And so, he said, "I am not worried at all about anything neurological with you, but I am worried about you having this baby and developing a walloping case of postpartum depression." And I didn't quite understand it, but I knew to fear it. I thought that postpartum depression involved feelings of wanting to hurt oneself or, much worse, the child. I knew that I had not experienced it the first time, despite some moments of blues or intense anxiety. But my two pregnancies were completely different.

As I sat in the neurologist's office, I listened as he dictated a memo to my obstetrician, urging him to pay attention to the gravity of my pain, both physical and emotional. I couldn't hear everything he said, though, as I was still lost under water, the words muffled as I floated down and down and down.

As my baby grew, and as his delivery grew closer, things got worse.

My numbness spread. My husband and I drifted. We each took our time dealing with our emotions, separately—divided. I continued to shut down and spiral. My husband did things to show me his love, to bring me back, but I was in a hole so dark that it was hard for me to see the light.

For the last two months of my pregnancy, I was experiencing painful Braxton Hicks contractions. The contractions were so strong that they would contort my entire belly into a strange shape, almost knocking me over. These moments of uncomfortable tightness would show up strongly on the hospital's fetal monitor. I went into the labor and delivery unit four times for "false alarms," as the contractions were present but not doing anything to induce real labor. My cervix was not softening, nor was I dilating. This came as no surprise to me, as I had never progressed more than one centimeter with my daughter, but the hospital staff seemed to be fixated on the numbers as opposed to the nuances of my case.

Because of my first cesarean section and the fact that my children don't seem to be able to engage my pelvis, I was scheduled for a repeat surgery on October 28, 2013. Not only was this a routine repeat, but my little boy, in all of his enormous glory, was lying in the transverse position inside of me. This means that instead of being head down (or, in breach cases, head up) he was lying smack across my stomach. I looked like I was smuggling a watermelon under my shirt. I was ridiculous looking. I was all belly, and my belly had a belly. I had mixed feelings leading up to my cesarean section. I was relieved, in some ways, to have the luxury of planning my second child's birth—to schedule a day and make sure that I had the proper preparations in place; to ensure that I said goodbye to my daughter meaningfully; to make sure that my nails and toes were perfect—but I was also scared. More than scared, I was terrified. I remembered the scary parts of my first C-section: the spinal and the feeling of not being able to breathe, only assuaged by the kind anesthesiologist who held a wet sponge to my parched lips, and then the whole "new baby" thing. I worried, every minute, about going through surgery, surviving surgery, and then surviving parenthood. I grew increasingly nervous as the date approached, and I spoke honestly to my husband, parents, friends, and obstetrician. My obstetrician would refer to the scheduled cesarean date as a "birthday party," while I looked at it as a day of dread. I was thinking catastrophically, sometimes drawing from my previous experience and sometimes having truly paranoid thoughts. And all of my "false alarm" trips to labor and delivery did nothing to ease my fears. In these times I had said, "See you soon, my love!" to my little Belle, adding, "We may be going to meet your brother!" and then had to waddle on out and come home hours later with a closed cervix and tons of embarrassment. And pain. And contractions. And, in one case, a sleepy baby.

Pregnancy didn't agree with me. And as much as I feared the next chapter and all that it meant, I was ready for a uterus eviction.

And then, at 4 a.m. on the morning of October 24, I awoke out of a dead sleep in pain. The kind of pain that is real, profound, where you can't really breathe and your stomach is tightening with pressure and pulsing. It was so painful that I woke up my husband. I was thirty-eight and a half weeks pregnant. My cesarean section was scheduled for the following Monday. And so, I said to myself, "Self. You are *not* going in again for a false alarm. You are not. If this means that you are having this giant transverse baby at home in your bathtub, so be it." I even went as far as to pack my daughter's lunch and included a note reading, "Four more days until you meet your baby brother!" I gave her a regular kiss goodbye. "See you after school!" I said.

By 10 a.m., when the contractions were becoming more painful and regular, and I was writhing in pain in my bed, I called my OBGYN. He asked me if these contractions felt different. And they did. And he told me I had to come in. "It may be party time!" he said. "If I feel any difference with your cervix, we will be having a birthday today!"

Oh, joy! My nails were chipped, my hair was dirty, and I had not said goodbye to my daughter. It could not be time. But the contractions were hurting so badly that I was nearly in tears. I called my mom.

"The doctor wants me to come in," I said sheepishly.

And, for the first time, her voice was different. "I think this is it," she said.

She arrived at my house in minutes. She supervised my shower, and we got ready to go.

For my other visits—my false alarms—I had been so sure that my delivery was imminent, but on this day, perhaps as a denial-based defense mechanism, I just kept repeating things like "This is ridiculous, why am I going in again, I am going to be pissed to be sent home again, blah da de blah blah!"

Because I was so skeptical, I didn't even tell my husband. I did, however, give my "on-call" friend a heads-up, in case we needed her to pick up my daughter from school. And, just in case, I wore my lucky underwear and purple socks, but I was still skeptical.

Upon our arrival at the hospital I was greeted as an old friend; everyone there knew me. The residents and I were on a first-name basis. It was embarrassing. But, I had to admit, the pain I was feeling was different. And the monitor showed the same. I was having strong contractions every three minutes, regularly.

But, alas, as has always happened when it comes to me and my labors, my cervix was not opening. Not at all. Not even one centimeter. So I waited in the bed, for hours, contracting to the point of agony, when I started to cry. I cried from the pain. I cried from the uncertainty. And, most of all, I cried because I hadn't said a proper goodbye to my daughter.

I had previously been having fantasies of how we'd spend our last night together as a tripod. We would have a special dinner, and then maybe

I'd sleep with her that night, since it would be our last time being just the three of us; I would sing in her ear and send her off to school with a special shirt.

But my son did not want to wait for our grand goodbye. He wanted to make an even grander hello. I was contracting and thinking and perseverating, and, all of a sudden, I started to cry again.

I cried to my mom, really from the pain, "I can't go another weekend like this." And I consider myself strong. Emotionally, I was most certainly a basket case, but, pain-wise, I am pretty darn tough. But I just knew, much like the first time around, that it was time for this baby to come out.

At about this time my OBGYN showed up. He confirmed what the residents had said, that my cervix was still closed, but added that it had softened a lot, and said that my contractions were really strong and regular on the monitor, inevitably putting stress on my uterus.

"Well, guess what? We are having a birthday party today!" he said.

And then I cried some more.

Out of relief, out of fear, and out of the "What the fuck?!" feeling of having planned everything, every last detail, and having it all turned upside down by a sideways (literally) baby.

And I still had not even called my husband.

At that point the doctor offered me an epidural to manage the pain until an operating room opened up, but I declined. If I could not experience a natural birth, which had been my dream, I would at least experience natural labor. And that I did. I am no masochist, but it made me feel like I could, at least, have some control over my body.

And so we called my friend once again to tell her that it was show time. She would watch my daughter and host a playdate with her son, whom Belle referred to as her "Prince Charming."

And then, finally, we called my husband. He was in a big meeting. He was told to rush out. He asked our nurse, over the phone, for permission to go home and change out of his suit. He was told that, no, he could not; there was no time.

I was forced to take off all of my clothes, including my lucky socks. And so when my husband arrived, handsome and dapper in his suit, I had him put on my lucky socks, in their neon purple glory, under his gray slacks and ultimately under his full scrub attire.

The next bit was a blur; I met with anesthesiologists, got an IV, and met my labor nurse. It was really happening. And my nurse, Katherine, held my hand and told me I'd be OK, as I told her how scared I was to go into surgery. How unprepared I felt. How my three-and-a-half-year-old needed me.

But then Katherine told me it was time. So my hair was placed in a net and I was placed in a wheelchair. I hugged my mom and husband tightly. It was time. I couldn't stop shaking. It was time.

Time to meet my son.

I arrived in the operating room and saw that, unlike the middle-of-the-night birth of my daughter, it was light outside, and I could see trees through the window. I was shaking uncontrollably, likely from adrenaline, and I asked every person I saw, from doctor to scrub tech, if I was going to die. They all assured me that I would be fine. For them, this was routine. For me, this was petrifying.

But despite these comforts and kind words, I could not stop shaking uncontrollably. A medical student called Doctor Anna hugged me and held me, telling me I was in good hands. She even continued to hug me as I had to curl my spine over in order to receive my epidural. After having explained my aversion to my previous spinal, the anesthesiologist decided to give me an epidural instead of the one-shot spinal, and it was a much slower onset, which I preferred greatly. They also gave me pain medicine and some anxiety meds through my IV, which the anesthesiologist equated to a glass of wine (as I did not want to feel too out of it but definitely needed to take the edge off).

At this point my OBGYN came in to "Get the party started! Woo!" and because an epidural works differently from a spinal, I could feel my body. I was not completely numb, nor disconnected from my lower half. I could feel so much that I heard them say, "Okay, it is time to insert the catheter," and I shouted, over the blue screen that they had put up between my face and surgical site, "I can still feel my vagina!"

The next part happened quickly: they opened me up; I smelled something strange (my burning, cauterized flesh); they told me that my husband (with his Day Glo socks) was allowed back into the operating room with me. My blood pressure kept dropping, I kept feeling scared, and I literally felt my entire body lift off the table as they yanked the baby out. I had not felt any of this the first time around, and it was strange and surreal.

I kept hearing them talking about things like seeing a hand and adhesions and blood, and I loved it and hated it all at once.

And then, all of a sudden, a cry. I had a son. And I looked at the clock.

My son was born at 4:11 p.m. April 11 is my birthday. For someone as superstitious as I am, this could not have been better. And, on the subject of numbers, my son came out weighing seven pounds, twelve ounces, which was the exact same weight as his sister, three and a half years earlier.

It is worth noting that he was seven pounds, twelve ounces at thirty-eight and a half gestational weeks, while she was full term at forty weeks, so apparently my uterus does indeed hand out an eviction to babies who are just that size. They were only a half inch apart, him being twenty-one and a half inches to her twenty-one inches. I make solid babies, it seems. I grow them, get them to a good size, and then my body says, "I am sorry, I will not open for you, but I will make sure that they know, quite clearly, that they are no longer welcome. Get out, babies. Get. Out."

And, because I had asked about it beforehand, they brought him to me, and I saw that he had fair hair and a cleft in his chin (like many of the men in my family), and I swear that when our faces touched he smiled.

Alexander Beau. We wanted our son to have a strong name, one that he could have as the president of the United States, an artist, a rock star, a doctor, or anything else—anyone else—that he came to be.

And then the world disappeared. I know that this sounds cliché or trite or like what I am supposed to say, but everything else melted away as my husband, son, and I cuddled up, as the doctors were still working to sew me up, and we sang to him. We held him and sang a song that my Pop Pop made up for us years ago:

> Mommy loves the baby,
> Daddy loves the baby,
> Everybody loves the little boy.

I do not remember when they took him away, but I do remember feeling as though the next stage of the "party" was taking an awfully long time. They had cut through many layers of my body, so I realized that they had to stitch me back, but it felt endless.

And then the warmth of having just delivered a perfect boy dissipated as the world started to turn black around me.

"I am going to pass out," I told the staff.

My blood pressure was continuing to drop. I was fading away. I now know that I was losing a large amount of blood.

Finally, I was sewn up. I was not made whole, but I was closed.

I recall so vividly desperately wanting to be out of the operating room and to hold my son, as I had not been able to hold my daughter. While they waited for a room to open up for us in the maternity ward, we were wheeled back into a labor and delivery room. Without having to wait too long, they brought my son in, all curled up in a swaddle blanket, looking tiny in his little plastic box. They handed him to me, I pulled down the side of my hospital gown to expose my breast, and he latched on immediately. I knew what I was doing and felt like a seasoned expert. It was so different, so much more pleasant than my first birth. I held him and nursed him, and I sent a text message to my best friends saying, "I have a son."

I had a son.

I can write honestly, despite it being hard, that the pregnancy with my son was not nearly as magical or enchanting as that with my daughter, but I must say, the birth and the time right thereafter was extraordinarily special.

But there was one milestone left to happen: we needed my daughter to meet her brother. She had been having a great time at her best friend's house, so much so that she peed her pants in all the excitement. I am proud to say that Belle met her baby brother for the first time wearing her boyfriend's cartoon-themed underpants and cargo pants. And, for some reason, a hat that looked like a panda's head.

At around six o'clock that evening, just an hour after my surgery had concluded, my little girl, who suddenly seemed so big, walked into the recovery room and over to her brother and said, "Hi, baby. I love you. Don't cry. Maybe I can carry him?"

And then there were four.

I will never, in all my life, forget the feeling of wholeness that that moment provided for me. All of my fears about not being able to love a second child, or a boy, washed away. I was instead swathed in rich, deep feelings of love and gratitude.

His birth and the hours postsurgery and the transition of my family from a triangle to a square happened seamlessly. It was not easy, but it was beautiful.

When he was born, I felt happy. I felt better. I remember telling this to a friend of mine, the hospital's nurse manager, when she came to visit me during her rounds. She surprised me by coming into our room with a blue balloon, and I apologized to her for having been so out of touch in the months prior.

"I don't know what was going on with me," I confessed. "I was so depressed. But now I feel so much better. I think I am finally better." And then I threw up into a bucket as she held back my hair.

I now know that my experience of perinatal distress is unique, and its presentation was atypical for several reasons: First, I had no preexisting mental health conditions. I did not have a history of depressive symptoms, which, as stated, is a major risk factor in developing both prenatal and postpartum depression. Second, I do not have a family history of perinatal mood disorders. Finally, my life situation during the time of my pregnancy would not be considered "unstable," and I had a very solid support system with my husband, family, and friends. Though my case is less common, many women do, in fact, have an unexpected onset of perinatal mood disorders during pregnancy, which is why I feel it is so salient that I share my honest story, and the stories of many others, in order to help current and future sufferers. My hard journey was not over, but there was hope on the other side.

5

❖ ❖

Violated Expectations of Magic

Dr. Amy Wenzel's Clinical Experience with Prenatal Distress

As mentioned, Dr. Amy Wenzel has written extensively on the subject of prenatal distress, from its onset through treatment options and beyond. Dr. Wenzel shared her clinical experience with me during our many meetings, emphasizing the importance of learning from her vast experience. While most of the research that we find—both as clinicians and as laypeople—is on postpartum depression and other postpartum mood disorders, Dr. Wenzel emphasizes the importance of educating people (women, caregivers, healthcare professionals, etc.) about what to do when a woman is pregnant and suffering. Postpartum depression has been talked about extensively in the media, which has served to destigmatize it—which is, of course, positive—but also, in some cases, to overshadow the very important care that women need during the prenatal period.

Dr. Wenzel says that even the research that is out there on prenatal mood disorders is limited. Generally, it is focused on one of two categories: medicine and preexisting depression. In regard to the former, there have been many studies done on women who take selective serotonin reuptake inhibitors (SSRIs), commonly known as antidepressants. This can be a controversial topic, as pregnant women are often leery of taking prescription medication, especially those medications that pose any risk to the fetus, no matter how small. "Of course you don't want to take medicine while pregnant," says Dr. Wenzel.

However, taking an SSRI is the classic case of risk versus reward; if a woman takes an SSRI that is deemed safe during pregnancy and breastfeeding, she is putting a chemical into her body, which can feel scary or unnatural. However, not treating a condition like depression can make a woman symptomatic, and therefore she may not engage in self-care. She may miss appointments with her doctor. She may not take the proper health precautions. Or she may experience an increase in cortisol, the stress hormone, which could be detrimental to both her and her unborn child. As counterintuitive as it may seem, oftentimes the use of SSRIs during pregnancy is more helpful than avoiding medication, which could lead to the onset or recurrence of depressive symptoms.

The latter area of study, involving preexisting depression, is not unrelated, but it also does not include the full scope of women who suffer from these prenatal mood disorders. As mentioned in this book, a woman can have no preexisting mental health conditions and a history of a mentally healthy postpartum period and still be afflicted with both prenatal and postpartum anxiety and depression. Though this situation may not be the statistical norm, it does happen, and therefore it should be documented, studied, and treated seriously.

Whether a pregnant woman has had preexisting mental health issues or is experiencing new feelings of distress during her pregnancy, she should consult with her psychiatrist as well as her obstetrician, ideally having them consult with one another, in order to form a treatment team to help her holistically. A pregnant woman is not just a belly, nor is she just a brain. Ideally, a collaborative treatment team can find a way to manage both the mother's mental health and the growing baby's care.

Dr. Wenzel has come across countless patients who have suffered from all forms of perinatal distress, with varying degrees of severity. Dr. Wenzel's patients span the spectrum in terms of having some sort of prenatal mood disorder, and in this chapter she shares six unique cases in which she has been able to help patients with various needs, degrees of severity in their symptoms, and outcomes.

In the six stories below, the names and identifying details of Dr. Wenzel's patients have been changed or omitted in order to keep private, sensitive information confidential and protected.

PATIENT STUDY 1

Dr. Wenzel treated a woman with obsessive compulsive disorder (OCD) both during and after pregnancy. After her first child was born, the woman was having intrusive thoughts obsessively—specifically that she had post-partum psychosis.

Dr. Wenzel explains that this woman did not, in fact, have postpartum psychosis, for three distinct reasons:

1. She had no prior history, nor any family history, of psychosis.
2. When these intrusive thoughts were occurring, the woman was ap-proximately six months postpartum, and postpartum psychosis would have happened much closer to the time that she had given birth.
3. Intrusive, dangerous thoughts would be ego-dystonic for this patient. As Dr. Wenzel explains, ego-dystonic anxieties are those that are not in line with one's values. Because her patient was so worried—ob-sessively so—about postpartum psychosis and its possible effects, it was evident that she would find that behavior disturbing, upsetting, or inconsistent with her identity. On the flip side, when something is ego-syntonic, a patient will feel comfortable with the behavior surrounding the condition or experience and treat it as though it is natural and acceptable.

A couple of years later, Dr. Wenzel's patient returned to treatment during a subsequent pregnancy, as she was suffering from a great deal of stress. As Dr. Wenzel explains, stress increases a person's vulnerability. This patient had stress in several areas of her life, including motherhood, marriage, and, most prominently, financial matters. She had to clean up messes every day, both literally and figuratively, and felt an extreme sense of burden. She and her husband each worked blue-collar jobs, so that when her husband was not working one of his many shifts, she would take the second shift at an overnight daycare.

And she could not sleep. Despite staying on her SSRI during this preg-nancy, the patient's intrusive thoughts, grueling work schedule, young tod-dler, and husband's excessive snoring all kept her up at night—all night, every night. She begged her psychiatrist for medication that would help her sleep, despite the contraindications. She would lament to Dr. Wenzel that she "would never sleep again" and believed her worrying thoughts. The patient became a zombie, trying to juggle so much stress.

Fortunately, once this patient had her baby, it was a relief to her and her family. She did not experience postpartum depression, despite her mental health issues during pregnancy. And, most important, she was able to sleep again.

PATIENT STUDY 2

This patient was referred to Dr. Wenzel while at the end of her first trimester, in an effort to help her with anxiety management. She was sent to Dr. Wenzel by her psychiatrist, who had been treating her for both low-level depression and low-level anxiety. At the time that Dr. Wenzel began seeing this woman, she was pregnant with her third child and had suffered from postpartum depression historically, which was why her psychiatrist felt that she would benefit from cognitive behavioral therapy (CBT) with Dr. Wenzel. In addition to the stress of pregnancy and her history with postpartum mood disorders, this patient had experienced significant marital problems after the births of her previous children.

After her previous pregnancy and marital strife, the patient had done therapeutic work with her husband, and their relationship had improved. When she started to see Dr. Wenzel, she did not have a specific pregnancy-related anxiety, but her relationship with her husband had taken a downward turn, despite their successful first course of treatment. Her husband was not supportive. The patient worked in the home all week, caring for her children and their house, and also worked outside of the home on weekends. Meanwhile, her husband did not carry his weight and would often say that they should not be having another child.

This patient described tremendous pressure from her husband to have sex, but she had a medical condition that made doing so very difficult for her. He was unsympathetic and insistent, even though she did not feel well or sexy. She worried that her husband would lose interest in her. She could not take care of her own needs, instead having to try to please him. In addition to his sexual demands, the patient's husband was not collaborative in their marriage in other ways, making unilateral decisions about their home and life. Generally, there was an uncomfortable home environment, and the idea that they would "not make it" as a couple was constantly looming, adding additional stress to an already tenuous situation.

With all that this woman had going on, it was hard for her to find the time to care for or worry about herself. However, she did develop one specific worry, as the baby was measuring large, which can be an indication of gestational diabetes.

While this patient's current status is unknown, her case is a very good example of how nature and nurture can interplay in a negative way during pregnancy. The combination of the woman's hormones with real-life stressors led to a prenatal mood disorder.

PATIENT STUDY 3

Dr. Wenzel also treated a pregnant woman who had a great deal of anxiety about the health of her unborn child. Though the woman had undergone procedures that screen for genetic diseases and abnormalities, which then ruled out these conditions, she could not assuage her fear that something would "be wrong" with her baby. Though the genetic screenings are approximately 99 percent accurate, Dr. Wenzel's patient ruminated that she would be the anomaly—the 1 percent—to have had a false negative report, and that the baby would be born with a condition or issue. This was her first pregnancy.

An interesting note about this patient, as Dr. Wenzel explains, is that she was so worried about her baby's health that it prevented her from being able to be sensitive or sympathetic to those around her. She had a sense of entitlement, expecting everyone around her to bend over backward in order to accommodate her anxiety. In the patient's mind, those around her should be very sensitive to her fears, and so her friends and family members had to walk on eggshells in order to avoid upsetting her.

To help her patient, Dr. Wenzel used both of the aspects that make up the practice of CBT: thoughts and behaviors. In terms of thinking, Dr. Wenzel tried to reorient this patient, reminding her of the data and facts that were being overshadowed by her fears. Not only had she had screenings done that were 99 percent accurate, but she was also very closely monitored during her pregnancy, making the likelihood of an unknown problem even smaller.

Most important, Dr. Wenzel worked with this patient on her behavior, which tied into her thoughts, by facilitating a sense of acceptance with her pregnancy and baby. Dr. Wenzel would reassure the woman that she would love her baby no matter what, prompting the woman to be exposed to her intrusive thoughts instead of neutralizing or invalidating them. Through their CBT work together, Dr. Wenzel helped this patient to manage her anxiety by giving her the tools with which to cope with the fears that had been crippling her.

PATIENT STUDY 4

This woman was a patient of Dr. Wenzel's when she accidentally became pregnant by her long-term partner. The patient had a history of depression, a major risk factor for perinatal mood disorders. Despite the pregnancy being unplanned, the woman married the father of her child and they decided to start a life together, buying a house that was far from Dr. Wenzel's practice. They would no longer be able to work together in person because of the distance.

Dr. Wenzel was committed to setting up her patient for success, and so she helped to facilitate a way for the pregnant woman to cope. Together, Dr. Wenzel and her patient made a "depression coping basket." In it, they carefully curated a collection of items, including chocolate, DVDs, CDs, and books that would serve to help her patient self-soothe in times of distress.

Though Dr. Wenzel would not be able to continue to treat this patient, the woman would be able to take a little piece of her psychologist with her, both tangibly and with all of the tools she had gained from their work together.

PATIENT STUDY 5

Dr. Wenzel is currently treating a patient with panic disorder. Her patient also has mild generalized anxiety and mild social anxiety. While her patient is not currently pregnant, she is getting married this year and is hoping to get pregnant soon thereafter.

Dr. Wenzel's concerns for her patient do not just stem from the fact that she suffers from anxiety-related disorders, as this woman has been taking medicine—on which she is dependent—for a very long time. With the presence of preexisting conditions being a major risk factor for future perinatal distress, along with this patient's plans to get pregnant, this could be a perfect storm, *especially* when trying to manage her brain chemistry with (or without) medication.

Additionally, this patient has a very demanding job as a nurse, and so she has little time for self-care. In her current state, this woman has difficulty coping with her anxiety and panic disorder, and so Dr. Wenzel worries about how she will be impacted by pregnancy, childbirth, and motherhood. She suffers from chronic fatigue, and pregnancy is likely to contribute to her exhaustion by (a) making it harder to sleep and (b) changing her hormones, which is why extreme exhaustion is a very common pregnancy symptom.

It is Dr. Wenzel's goal, through compassionate care, to cope ahead with her patient, in order to set her up for success. Knowing that the patient is at risk for prenatal distress and postpartum depression, Dr. Wenzel will employ the aforementioned holistic approach, by giving her CBT tools and working with her psychiatrist to determine the best course of action with her medication. It is her hope that by planning in advance and laying the groundwork of support, she can help her patient to have a pregnancy with minimal distress.

PATIENT STUDY 6

Dr. Wenzel recently started to treat a patient who felt as though Dr. Wenzel's unique areas of expertise would be a "great match for the specific anxieties" that she was suffering from most acutely. The patient was eager for help, which can be a great predictor for success, and when she initially contacted Dr. Wenzel, she explained that she had read several of her books. Though this woman lived in a different county, she was willing to make the commute to see Dr. Wenzel for treatment, as her anxiety had gotten out of control. She wanted help.

Dr. Wenzel's patient was looking to become pregnant for the second time and had a diagnosis of OCD. The patient explained that she had previously suffered with OCD for ten years, but it had been at its worst during her prenatal periods. She had a toddler-aged son. She also suffered from severe prenatal anxiety with her son, compounded by the fact that he was conceived after a miscarriage. It is Dr. Wenzel's assertion that women who have suffered from a pregnancy loss are at a much higher risk for prenatal distress, as they have been conditioned to worry about "something going wrong."

Dr. Wenzel's patient had been trying to conceive for a long time and suffered a second miscarriage after her healthy live birth two and a half years prior. Not only was she suffering from obsessive tendencies, but she was also stressed about getting pregnant and staying pregnant. She was concerned that she would not be able to conceive another healthy baby and simultaneously scared about what the pregnancy would look and feel like for her, after two losses and a viable pregnancy that was rife with stress and fear. This woman was so fearful about a future pregnancy that she was ambivalent about moving forward with her efforts in trying to conceive; she described it herself as being "at a crossroads." She did not want her fears to dominate her, stopping her from expanding her family, but at the same time she was desperate for help from Dr. Wenzel.

Dr. Wenzel's decision to take on this new patient was informed by her confidence in the fact that she could help to manage the woman's existing OCD and anxiety, set up coping mechanisms during the conception process, and continue to help to treat these afflictions and any other perinatal mood disorders should she become pregnant. Dr. Wenzel's keen awareness of the risk factors for prenatal and postpartum mood disorders would allow them to cope, using CBT and other therapeutic tools, and she could work holistically with her treatment team in order to ensure the best outcome for the mother and baby, before, during, and after pregnancy.

IN SUMMARY

Prenatal mood disorders can occur at any time before or during pregnancy, for women who are first-time mothers or experiencing their tenth pregnancy, in those patients with a family history, personal history, pre-existing conditions, or no risk factors at all. Some women can be treated by simply coping ahead, while others need to be medicated; there are a spectrum of severity and an array of treatment options available for those pregnant women who are struggling. The patient case studies shared above illustrate just how different each case of prenatal distress (particularly with anxiety and depression as a focus) can be. However, despite many external differences, each of the patients that Dr. Wenzel has treated or is treating currently shares one common connection: suffering. Each woman wants the best for herself and for her future family. Each woman has sought help for her afflictions and has chosen to do so with an expert in the field of perinatal mood disorders. Dr. Wenzel's patients have made the decision to fight against their mental health conditions in order to cope, survive, and thrive. Dr. Wenzel uses a positive attitude, a holistic approach to healing, and she treats each patient as an individual while also recognizing the commonalities that exist among all perinatal mood disorder sufferers.

6

❖ ❖

"I See the Light Going Out in Your Eyes"

The Beginning of My Postpartum Depression

After giving birth to my son, whom we called Beau, I felt an initial high. It was magical. He would sleep next to me on our small hospital bed, and we fit, so effortlessly, and it felt right. I was content and felt happy and blessed.

Our first days in the hospital were pleasant ones, as I felt savvy in my ability to breastfeed with ease, competent in knowing how to hold and burp a baby, and honored to be able to say the words "my son." The darkness that I had been experiencing had lifted, giving way to a warm glow of love, encompassing our new family.

On the third day postpartum, something changed. The change was so palpable that even the hospital room looked different to me, as if I had been transported somewhere else. That was the day that I was "in the other room," which, to this day, I cannot explain. Every single thing about the world appeared different. What I did not know at the time was that I had lost a lot of blood during my complicated cesarean section. I had a ghostly white pallor to my face, and the glow started to fade, until it morphed into pure sallowness. I was put through tests and my heart was constantly monitored for acute tachycardia.

Though I was still experiencing happiness, the ghosts that had haunted me throughout my pregnancy began to creep back into my head, with negative thoughts weaving through the channels in my brain like poison.

I was given the hospital's standard screening for postpartum depression. I failed. The questionnaire had instructed me to most closely rate my feelings, answering questions on a scale from zero to three, based on my mood in the seven days prior to taking the examination. The questions were about my ability to feel happy, the frequency that I was feeling anxious or sad, and whether I was having trouble sleeping. Though my memory of this test is vague, I remember indicating that I had not felt happy; had been experiencing trouble sleeping; and, due to intrusive thoughts, had been crying excessively and was scared. To put it in blunt terms, I was not OK. Though a social worker came to visit me to go over my results, she simply recommended that I seek help if needed and went about her day. I was not flagged as a danger to myself or to others. I did spend unplanned extra time in the hospital, but this was because of the blood that I had lost during my surgery, not because I was in a mental health crisis. After an additional two days in the hospital, I went home, with my husband, baby boy, and mounting fears and anxieties.

In the beginning of November, a week after my son's birth and my major abdominal surgery, I started to crumble. There was a part of me that was self-aware enough to think that something was wrong. It was not like the "case of the blues" that I had experienced after the birth of my daughter. The sadness felt ominous, like a storm I could see on the horizon—black, swirling clouds moving steadily in my direction.

I went from being more sad than happy to being only sad and never happy. I tried to hide it. My insides were fighting demons, and I wanted to win. The poison continued to seep through my brain; it infiltrated every part of me.

Though I didn't know exactly what postpartum depression was, I knew that it could sometimes lead to a mother wanting to hurt her child. For me, that was never the case. None of my depressed feelings had to do with my children. In fact, I was not even overwhelmed by having two kids. I was never resentful of them, and I certainly never wanted to do anything but love them. I did not wish to harm them in any way. I was lucky in that regard, as, for some women, the disease manifests itself differently, tragically.

All of the feelings of anger, loathing, sadness, and hatred were focused on me. Yet I still tried to hide it. It was too scary to even broach.

At the end of that first week in November, as I was finishing up a nursing session with my son, I got a text message from my husband. It read, "Just checking in on you. I want to make sure you're OK. I see the light starting to go out in your eyes."

I held my phone like it was my lifeline; if I could hold on to that phone, then I could hold it all together. And when my hand shook so badly that the phone fell from my grasp, I started to sob. I sobbed because I was so loved. I sobbed because I knew that he was right.

It was then, two weeks after giving birth, that I decided to seek therapy for my symptoms. I was tired and grumpy with a short fuse. I was sad and weepy, no longer able to find any joy in the things that had once made me happy.

And then there were the worse things. I thought about my life a lot and why it was worth living. *If* it was worth living. I knew, intellectually, that it was, but it was hard to feel it.

My therapist diagnosed me with postpartum depression and prescribed medicine for me to take. Taking this medicine would mean that I would have to wean my son, and I refused. Because I had breastfed my daughter for eighteen months, breastfeeding was a part of my identity as a mother. So, as an alternative, I tried talk therapy and additional childcare support, but it was clear that these measures were not enough. I was in a dark place, and the hormones, chemicals, and lack of sleep were proving to be a toxic combination for my body and my brain.

I started to face some resistance from my loved ones and my professional team. My symptoms were getting worse. I was sad, scared, and scaring those around me. I was tired all of the time, but I could not sleep. I loved my baby viscerally, but it felt hard to bond in the way that I had so easily with my daughter. My bad moments were getting more frequent, my good moments were scarce, and a cocktail of strong medicine was recommended by my psychiatrist.

Once again I was told that by agreeing to take the medication, I would have to also agree to give up breastfeeding. Someone told me, "It is better for your son to have a mom without a boob than a boob without a mom," but it was still too hard for me. I kept on nursing and kept on going down a spiral of deep, deep depression.

More people started to notice my state of suffering around Thanksgiving. It was the holiday that I had always cherished the most, and yet I spent that Thanksgiving in the corner of my aunt's living room, speaking to no one, falling asleep in the corner, on the arm of a big leather chair. Instead of letting him be held and admired by my loved ones, I insisted upon keeping my one-month-old son in his car seat next to me. I was so out of it that I did not even recognize how different my behavior had become; something that would have normally been the source of shame just felt like a necessity. I had to sleep. It did not matter when or where or how inappropriate. I needed to rest my troubled mind. Turkey did not stand a chance against torment.

I was withdrawing from my friends. They would call and leave messages or offer to drop off food, and I could not reply. I would like to say that this was an effort to hide my pain, as I was supposed to be feeling happy, but there was nothing conscious about my reclusiveness. I became quiet in my online presence, shunning the blog that I had worked so hard to build for over two years. I was slipping away.

And then things got worse. A lot worse. The feelings that I had been having about my life and its meaning started to take over me like a demonic plague. I couldn't think rationally. I could not feel happiness or love. All that I could feel was pain. The world—once so colorful to me— had turned black and cold. The storm was drawing closer. I could feel the wind, the air, swirling violently. I could imagine the pelting of the rain, and I did not know whether I wanted to be hit.

Until I did. I knew. I believed that I would feel better if I could feel the pain of the hail and the ice and the cold. And if I did not feel it emotionally, I would make sure to feel it physically.

This is one of the hardest things for me to share, as it takes me and my story to a new place. A much darker place. In writing about it, I feel a mix of sadness, incredulity, and shame. I am not sure exactly how it started, but it was at this time that I began to self-mutilate. This period of time was the first and only time in my life thus far during which I would engage in self-harm, further illustrating the fact that I was not myself, but rather completely corrupted and overcome by my postpartum depression.

At first, I used my necklace to inflict harm. When my grandparents were married for forty years, my Pop Pop designed a necklace for my Mom Mom. It is in the shape of two diamond hearts, each with a stone inside: a sapphire for my aunt's birthstone and an emerald for my mom's. It is a pin, strung on a necklace. This necklace became a family tradition and each woman, when they reached a milestone birthday, received a copy of this same necklace.

And so I would open it up, take the sharp point of the pin, and press it into the flesh of my left outer forearm. I was not slitting my wrist; I was drawing lines. Graffiti, like I once traced happily in the sand at the beach with my then-boyfriend. Within a week my arm became a mangled mess, torn up by the pin, my nails, and any sharp objects that I could find: tweezers, small bathroom scissors, and even my husband's razor blade, used cautiously. I had become a tormented street artist, using my frail, pale arm as my canvas, coloring it in shades of bright red and pink and brown scabs.

It was mid-December, six weeks after my son was born, and it was my sister's twenty-fifth birthday. I had always given her perfume for special gifts, helping her to choose a signature scent, and so I went to the fanciest department store in our area to test out the fragrances. I brought a friend with me, not just for her taste and guidance but also because I only had one usable wrist on which to test the scents. My left arm was untouchable, and I had to wear special, long-sleeved shirts with thumbholes in order to hide my wounded arm. It was horrifying to look at, and spraying perfume on it would have been agonizing, though, thinking back on it, I am sure that I would not have minded the pain. I simply did not want to make others uncomfortable. I had become unrecognizable to myself. An other.

I had done research on perfumes before our trip to Saks Fifth Avenue and thought that I would be getting Tom Ford's "Black Orchid," but when I smelled it I realized that it was not right, and so I tried out every one of Bond No. 9 New York's fragrances, each named for an area in New York City. At the time, my sister was living downtown and working as a journalist, so it seemed fitting to choose "Chinatown," with notes of peach blossoms, gardenia, tuberose, patchouli, and cardamom. It smelled fresh and cool and a bit dark and musky, and so, confident in my selection, I bought my sister a special and extravagant gift, feeling almost like a person.

After the salesman rang me up and we arranged everything so that the gift would be shipped to my sister's New York address, the salesman told me that I had to try one of their Central Park scents, and so he took my left arm in his hand and began to lift my shirt to expose my wrist. I saw lines of bright, angry red peeking out and pulled my hand away in horror.

"Thank you so much," I choked. "I have a signature scent that is very 'me,' so I am good for now, but I will definitely be back!"

He handed me a bag of samples, my friend gave me a hug, and I tugged the sleeve of my shirt down as far as it would go, almost covering my whole left hand.

The mutilation and my deterioration continued and worsened over the next week.

In order to ensure my safety, my family members had to stay with me at all times, taking shifts so that I was never left alone. My therapist privately reached out to my husband. She told him that I needed to be hospitalized. I needed specialized treatment for postpartum depression, and I needed it urgently. I was a suicide risk. She found a specific postpartum program in another state, affiliated with Brown University. She, as much as everyone else who cared for me, feared for my safety deeply.

I was not given any real choice in the matter. Though I was not committed involuntarily, I was also not a functional human being, but rather a shell. At that point I was either crying or a zombie, so, in my haze, I made a phone appointment and plans to check in to the recommended postpartum treatment center, one in which I could keep my son with me. I would keep nursing and try to recover before it got worse. I was catching this when it was still "stage one," to—with great sensitivity—liken my mental illness to a familiar way of categorizing similarly lethal physical afflictions. While this is not a clinical diagnosis, it is a metaphor that seemed apt. At this stage, I would be able to keep breastfeeding. I spoke to the intake coordinator at Brown and clearly met all criteria for admission; the problem was getting a spot. I could be admitted if I started the next business day, but if I could not get there—to Rhode Island from Philadelphia—soon enough, then I would have to wait at least another month until a new spot opened up.

This made the decision to go tremendously hard. I did not want to leave my daughter, especially with no notice. I felt every emotion from ashamed to terrified. I weighed my options; assessed the severity (to the extent that I could) of my condition; and, because my doctor and family members were essentially forcing me, said I would go to the treatment center.

I would be uprooting our lives, just because I was suffering, and so the guilt hit me and continued to rain down on me like a painful deluge. I had to pack for my husband, my baby son, and myself, and I had to get everything situated at home for my daughter. I felt crazed as I scrambled to get ready, as I ruminated on the fact that I was about to travel many hours with my husband and son, leaving my daughter with my parents, without any notice or time to prepare. It was a blur. My husband took me out to get the necessary supplies while my parents watched the kids.

But then I did something strange. I insisted on going out to the movies. We saw *American Hustle* in a crowded theater, and my phone buzzed the entire time with calls from the head physician at Brown and follow-up calls and texts from my own psychiatrist asking, "Where are you?" and demanding, "You need to answer. This is very time sensitive."

Perhaps I was in denial. Perhaps, somewhere deep inside me, I thought that if I focused on watching Bradley Cooper and Jennifer Lawrence and the figures dancing before me on the giant screen in the dark room, I wouldn't actually have to go away. Perhaps a part of me thought that if I pretended that life was normal, it would go back to being normal, and that the postpartum depression would end, along with the movie's rolling credits.

Instead, I just upset my psychiatrist, and my husband spent half of the movie speaking to her from the hallway outside of the theater. Guilt, guilt all around.

We got home from our errands and the movie when the sky had already turned dark and I saw my parents sitting in the living room with my kids. My mom held my baby as I went over to him and kissed him.

He was hot.

He was burning up.

Things were going from heated to hellish. Fire licked at my feet as I buried my head into my son's skin, tears beginning to form in my eyes.

The closer I got to him, the hotter he felt.

Hell. I had landed in hell.

7

❖ ❖

A Bicycle Built for Two (If That Bicycle Were Actually an ER Suite)

My Severe Postpartum Depression

As I pressed my cheek against my son's head, and then his stomach, I felt intense heat emanating from his soft skin. I undid his long-sleeved, one-piece bodysuit and felt his stomach. More heat. I took him upstairs and set him on the soft muslin changing pad cover.

I took his temperature, and it was 100.4, the magic number for a baby under two months old. He was just three days shy of his two-month birthday. It was a Saturday. Our pediatrician's office was closed. We had to take him to the hospital.

At my own darkest moment, I had a sick baby for whom to care. At the emergency room they gave him urgent care immediately. I can remember the triage room, and I remember being so scared. They tried to put a monitor that looked like a cloth bandage on his little toe and it wouldn't stay on. He cried. I cried.

We were brought back to a private room immediately, and we were never without a member of the medical team.

Once the staff pediatrician saw us, she explained that they had to do a full septic workup, including a complicated blood draw, a catheterization, and, worst of all, a spinal tap. This took three tries. To get an IV into his chunky little arm, they had to use a light that looked like a laser pointer to find his veins. It was all so alien, and surreal. And scary. Terrifying.

His blood oxygen level was low, and he had monitors all over him. One of the tests performed was a nasal swab. From this, he was diagnosed with respiratory syncytial virus (RSV), which had presented itself in my daughter as a cold earlier in the week. I knew about RSV, as my daughter had suffered from it at two and three years old, and for her it was a bit scary and a huge pain. We had to nebulize her with a steroid mist, and the noise of the loud breathing machine and the mask she had to wear made it nightmarish for her. When the doctor gave me my son's diagnosis, I felt myself hating those three letters more than I could have ever imagined.

And then, moments after his diagnosis was presented, while standing beside his bed in the ER, out of sheer stress and malnourishment, I passed out. I had to be admitted. My son and I spent a cold night in December in adjoining rooms of the emergency room, each hooked up to tubes, each receiving a myriad of tests, and each fighting.

They took my pulse and my blood pressure and my blood and gave me three bags of IV fluids.

"Do you ever have any thoughts of hurting yourself?" asked the nurse.

"I am dealing with severe postpartum depression," I told her.

She made sure that I was being cared for by a doctor and, although I did not always feel safe, that I was, in fact, safe.

I was in a stretcher, tethered to my IV pole, but I could see the form of my son from across the adjoining space.

He looked so tiny in the adult-sized bed across the long, double room. I couldn't reach out and touch him; I was hooked up to too many wires and tubes pumping me with saline in an attempt to raise my blood pressure. I remember the nurse handing me a potassium pill, since my blood tests showed a deficiency.

I needed help.

After another hour in our suite—the least glamorous "suite" of my life—we were told that my son would be admitted to the pediatrics floor of the hospital. His blood oxygen was still not where they wanted it to be, despite the steroids and oxygen in his nose.

My son needed more help, around the clock, and so he was checked in and brought up to a room and hooked up to more tubes in another too-big bed.

My baby boy spent four days in the hospital. At first he was released, since his blood oxygen level had improved, but we had to bring him back to the ER after a few hours at home. During the time we spent in our house, we noticed that he was breathing heavily and laboriously. He was experiencing stridor, a noisy, high-pitched breathing that created a wheezing sound. We could see his stomach suck in involuntarily and violently, his rib cage exposed as he desperately tried to find air.

It was in the hospital that first night that he was given his first bottle of formula. It was in the hospital that first night that I began to take the medicine I needed.

I was placed on an antidepressant, an antianxiety medication, and a mood stabilizer. I had a very bad reaction to the last drug, a side effect called akathisia. That is the technical name, but I felt as though I were crawling out of my skin. My son had been admitted to the hospital, but I was not the one staying with him, caring for him, calming him, holding him, or soothing him. I would go for short visits, and because I felt an insufferable restlessness in my limbs, I would hop around, stretch, and lie down, my body contorted.

As I raced in and out of that hospital room—and, for the record, the saddest place in the world to be during Christmastime is the children's ward of a hospital—I saw my baby, so tiny, hooked up to tubes, with oxygen in his nose. He was like a bird, a nest of worn, threadbare swaddling blankets from the hospital surrounding him, but he didn't have his mama bird to shield him with her wing or to put worms into his mouth with her own. His mama was flying around in circles, not knowing where to land, but flapping away, relentlessly, mercilessly.

It began to work. For both of us, it began to work.

Since the winter of 2013 I have been in treatment for mental health issues that I did not have prior to the conception of my son earlier that year. My official diagnoses are anxiety, depression, post-traumatic stress disorder (PTSD), and what my doctor calls an unspecified feeding disorder, as my depression and the side effects of some of the medications have caused me to lose weight; I am considered "clinically malnourished." This is different from an eating disorder, like anorexia or bulimia, in that I do not have a distorted body image, restrict calories, or purge my food; rather, I have a hard time actually taking in the food that I need in order to be physically and mentally healthy. I take an antianxiety medicine and an antidepressant, have been on and off a mood stabilizer, and, at one point, was even given a blood pressure medicine (despite my already low blood pressure) in order to help me with the debilitating nightmares that I was having six times a week. Apparently, doctors found that if they gave this blood pressure medication to soldiers who had fought in Afghanistan, it helped them with their PTSD symptoms, and it also helped with mine.

My road has not been a straight one, though I believe I have traveled toward healing. There have been dips and some backsliding, but I am a healthier person, in general, than I was three years ago.

I have engaged in traditional talk therapy with psychologists, psychiatrists, and social workers. I have seen a family therapist as a way to bolster my support system at home. I have seen a couple's therapist in order to help my husband and me through this arduous time and to try to get past the trauma of what we have endured. I have done some cognitive behavioral therapy (CBT) and worked extensively in a program that focuses on one of its offshoots, dialectical behavioral therapy (DBT). My work with DBT involved individual counseling with a psychologist and a group that would meet for several hours a week, during which time we learned about tools in the areas of interpersonal effectiveness, mindfulness, emotion regulation, and distress tolerance.

In an effort to help with my weight issue, I have been through many courses of treatment. In the fall of 2014 I was hospitalized at Princeton Hospital, first as an outpatient, and then admitted for an inpatient stay, in order to help with the refeeding process. This, however, was a challenge, as I do not suffer from a traditional eating disorder and therefore do not need that type of therapy. I just need to be fed.

I have worked in other outpatient treatment centers—solely for the meals—but haven't found them to be a good fit. I have worked with a medical doctor who was very focused on the numbers on the scale, and I realized that the medical weight avenue was not a good one for me. My soul needed mending before those numbers would start to creep back up. For a couple of years now I have worked with an amazing, kind, patient registered dietician. We focus on my limitations, meal planning, and life coping skills, and I still have weekly weigh-ins. She is a confidant, a steadfast supporter. I am sure that she will help me gain weight again when my body is ready for it. Sometimes, I have learned, the mind heals first, and then the body will follow.

I spend many, many hours a week in therapy, either directly or doing work outside of the office in order to improve my health and my life.

But there is still one issue: the hardest part.

I can no longer have children.

I am always careful when addressing this part of my story, as it is one of the most sensitive issues, not only for me but also for many others. Let me say that I am incredibly, indescribably grateful that I have my two children. I have a daughter. I have a son. I grew them with my own body and carried them, birthed them, and nursed them. I had two pregnancies, both challenging in their own ways, both certainly different, but each with at least a bit of magic. I had two cesarean sections that were scary and, at times, a bit precarious, but my surgeries produced babies with Apgar scores of eight and then nine.

I felt the magic. And so I know how lucky I am. And that magic is what I mourn the most.

You see, there is nothing like that magic. And, once again, please know that I am writing this with the utmost sensitivity and also with my own perspective, one that is, undoubtedly, biased. For me, there is nothing like finding out that there is life growing inside of you. There is nothing like the first flutters that feel like the flapping of a butterfly's wing. There is nothing like seeing the first ultrasound. There is nothing like finding out the baby's sex and coming up with names and imagining what the person, burrowed so deep inside, will look like. There is nothing like the unknown last days. There is nothing like the drive to the hospital. The anticipation. There is nothing like hearing "This is it!" and there is absolutely nothing like seeing the baby for the first time. Those first few moments, and then days. The hospital stay (which, after baby number one, seems luxurious).

And the loss of that, of knowing I will never have that incredible feeling ever again, is what makes me feel sad.

Sometimes I anticipate the sadness. If I am going to visit a friend's new baby or put my arms around a best friend's pregnant belly, I can expect to feel the pang. But, as I have come to realize, this is why I have two hands—not just literally but also figuratively. In some ways, it is the epitome of dialectical thinking. In those moments I feel so much joy for my friends. It is genuine. It is not about me at all. In one of my hands I carry nothing but happiness. And then there are other times, times when I'm unarmed, when my armor is off, that I feel the pain so deeply it is almost hard to breathe. The wind gets knocked out of me. In my other hand, I carry my pain.

I want to be completely transparent here in that I am extremely sensitive to the fact that many people cannot have children, for myriad reasons, and that I feel lucky to have two. I do not take that for granted in any way, nor do I lack sympathy or compassion. My sadness comes from the fact that the choice was taken from me, and at twenty-eight years old I was told that it would no longer be safe for me to have more children, as my body and brain would likely turn against me. By that I mean that my abdomen is filled with scar tissue and my uterus is now thinner, putting me at a higher risk for a rupture, which could, in the worst-case scenario, endanger not only the life of a fetus but also my own life. Psychologically, having suffered from the severe perinatal distress, I am now at a much greater risk for suffering from that affliction again. I survived last time—both physically and emotionally—but a future pregnancy could kill me. That is not hyperbolic or melodramatic; it is just the truth. A very hard truth, but the truth nonetheless.

Months ago, when I went up to our playroom to pick up after my kids, I got walloped. I was cleaning up tutus and dresses and toy cars when I saw a hand-sewn pillow among a pile of dress-up clothing. This pillow is a bit threadbare and, if I am being honest, not exactly my style, but it is in the shape of a heart and was given to me by my weekend nurse, Pam, when I had my son. Pam assisted me when it was still too hard for me to stand after my surgery. She told me to press the pillow into my incision when I would try to move, and that the pressure against my incision would relieve some of the pain.

When I saw that pillow, tears came to my eyes.

I will never have that feeling again.

It happens when I go to a doctor's appointment at the hospital. I still see some specialists at the hospital where I gave birth to both of my children. The hospital, for me, is haunted. When I drive into the garage I picture myself, just a few years ago, walking through the darkness, cradling my giant belly in my hands.

I enter the building and walk past the outpatient lab. I can't help but look inside and I instinctively picture myself twelve weeks pregnant, feeling shocked by the unexpected information at our sequential screen ultrasound when the tech told us that he saw "something between the baby's legs." It was in that lab that I called my dad and told him that we were having a boy.

When I need to, I walk with trepidation over to the medical office building and take the elevator, the same elevator that I rode every month, and then every week, to check on my babies' heartbeats while they were still inside of me. That is where my OBGYN's office is located. I see the countless figures in scrubs and they become a blur to me, a sea of what I can't have. Sometimes it is OK, and sometimes, in that sea, I feel myself drowning.

Being in the hospital hurts.

Because I am of childbearing age, I have to tell people quite often that I will no longer be bearing any children of my own. It comes up at the most random of times, and it ranges from a passing comment to slightly awkward to downright unpleasant. I have to tell doctors and nurses, especially when I am being given a new medicine or scheduling a procedure. I seem to have to tell people every time I am pushing a child or two in a stroller around the town. I say it to the people at my children's schools. Sometimes it is met with skepticism: "Oh, well, you never know," with a sly smile.

But I know.

I have grown a team.

I get to sing the beautiful, classical lullabies and mean every word, so deeply, that my bones tingle and my heart aches.

But, despite all of that, it is still hard. Just as this time in my life has been hard.

That magic, while powerful, is also connected to something that scares the people who love me the most. It is not that they do not want me to have another baby; they are just frightened for me, both for my body and for my brain.

And not everyone understands my struggle. During this time in my life I have lost friends, friends whom I thought would be true to me forever. I have scared my family members, and I have upset my children when they have seen me curl up or cry. I have lost weight and lost color in my face, and still I cannot get over this idea that, despite all of these things, I am out of control of my own body, mind, and future.

Sometimes I put a positive spin on things, and I think about how I am now forever done with the exhausting newborn phase and how my two children are both healthy and strong, and I feel so glad that I will not have another scary cesarean section surgery.

But there is this part of me, this small part, that still grieves. Because there is this little part of me that thinks that there is this little baby out there that I will never know. That it should exist. And that I'm missing it.

I will never feel the magic again. I don't have a choice, and I won't have the chance.

I will see my son squirm around before me and say, without thinking, "This is exactly what he used to do in my stomach, remember?" And then I will say, "I will never feel that again."

There are different stages of grief. Perhaps my belief that there is a baby out there waiting for me is denial.

Sometimes I have dreams that the doctor was wrong, that I can, actually, decide to "try" again. I can wait, with a quickened heartbeat, for two lines to appear on a stick. I can see a tiny teddy bear–shaped person flickering on an ultrasound. I can find out if the baby is a boy or a girl. I can feel kicks and feel nauseated and feel the baby being pulled from inside of me as I hear the doctor say, "I see a hand! I see a foot!"

Sometimes I feel angry, at my body and at my brain chemistry and at my doctors. I am angry that this happened to me.

Other times I ask my husband if, in six years, assuming we have loads of money, we could hire a surrogate to carry a third baby for us. Bargaining.

And then there's the depression. The part of me that is making my eyes sting now as I type these words.

I am waiting for the acceptance.

But until I find it, which I pray that I do, I will go on rooting for my team. The shop is closed.

So for now I will enjoy my babies and appreciate them more than they will ever know. I will celebrate the births of my friends' children. And I will try to exorcise the ghosts when I walk through the hospital halls.

My shop is closed. But there is great joy ahead. There are memories to be made, milestones to face, dance parties to have, hands to hold, and heartbeats to listen to. There are lullabies to sing and lives to live.

My shop is closed, but so, so many doors have yet to be opened.

FROM PERSONAL INTERVIEWS WITH DR. WENZEL

Perinatal distress is depression or anxiety during pregnancy and the postpartum period.

The postpartum period is defined as being the first four weeks following childbirth. However, most experts say that the postpartum period is the first year following childbirth.

Despite the fact that many people classify postpartum depression as being unique, putting it in its own category, it actually has many of the same characteristics as any other kind of depression.

There are nine characteristics of general clinical depression:

1. Having a depressed mood more of the time than not
2. Loss of interest or pleasure in activities that one would typically find enjoyable and pleasurable
3. Appetite disturbance (overeating or undereating)
4. Sleep disturbance (trouble sleeping or sleeping excessively)
5. Psychomotor disturbance (the state of being agitated or fidgety) or psychomotor retardation, which is when one is moving more slowly than what is normal
6. Lack of energy or fatigue

7. Sense of worthlessness or excessive and inappropriate guilt
8. Difficulty concentrating or indecisiveness
9. Suicidal ideation (thoughts that life is not worth living)

The differences between general depression and postpartum depression are, however, highlighted as such:

1. Postpartum depression can be very abrupt.
2. There is a newborn child who needs care, and so a woman and the people around her are concerned about caring for the child.
3. Becoming a mother carries such significant meaning that when the experience does not go exactly the way that one expects it to go, it can be absolutely devastating.

Risk factors for postpartum depression include prenatal distress and depression or anxiety during pregnancy.

The "intolerance of uncertainty" is currently getting a great deal of attention in the field of psychology. The "intolerance of uncertainty" represents one example of how different cognitive styles can impact a woman's likelihood for developing perinatal distress, including postpartum depression. Most people, of course, do not like uncertainty, but if a person is already characterized by that psychological trait, meaning that she has more anxiety about the unknown than what is considered "typical," then pregnancy will pose a great challenge, as pregnancy is completely uncertain. There are other cognitive behavioral traits that are risk factors for prenatal distress. An example of one of these qualities is if a person struggles with perfectionism or has rigid expectations. Another character trait is called "overestimation of responsibility," which means that if a woman is naturally one to put a lot of pressure on herself or duties on her plate, then she is at a higher risk of developing an issue. These are obsessive compulsive disorder (OCD) traits.

Under the OCD umbrella there are two other noteworthy risk factors: morality bias and probability bias. Morality bias occurs when a woman believes that the act of thinking something negative makes her a bad person. Probability bias occurs when a woman believes that if she has a negative thought, then there is a high likelihood that she will act on that thought.

One of the most difficult aspects of diagnosing postpartum depression is that so many normal struggles that are attributed to anyone with a newborn can appear to fit (at least some of the) criteria for clinical depression listed above. One of the reasons why this diagnosis can be challenging is that the symptoms manifest differently in every woman and can be confused by extenuating situations and lurking variables. For example, in trying to evaluate a woman's appetite or sleep, it is almost impossible to do so accurately when she is taking care of a newborn. This example is highlighted in terms of sleep disturbance. It is commonly accepted that newborns require round-the-clock care, thus disrupting normal sleep patterns. A sign of a problem, however, is if a woman is not able to rest when her baby is resting. Another apt example is the so-called baby blues that up to 80 percent of woman experience in the week following their delivery. A way to distinguish normal postpartum stress from true postpartum depression is if problems like sadness and anxiety persist. If a woman appears to be particularly tearful, it could be a physiological issue, hormonal fluctuation, or emotional expectation.

One risk factor for postpartum depression is when a woman has rigid expectations for what motherhood should be like. For example, a woman may have preconceived notions about breastfeeding, and if she is having lactation problems, she may assume that she will not be able to bond with her baby in the same way that she would if she were nursing. Another example is if a woman plans to have a vaginal birth and ends up needing a cesarean section. Because the birth did not go as planned, she may be plagued with guilt. Many postpartum depression sufferers feel that they are "less of a woman" because they failed to live up to their rigid expectations. Some women believe they are "less of a mother" if they did not go through the "rite of passage" of vaginal birth.

Women who are not functioning well may be suffering from postpartum depression. However, there are many variables to consider when determining whether a woman is not functioning. New mothers may not feel physically well or may not be sleeping properly, for example. When a woman's failure to function is considered above a moderate level, she may be suffering from postpartum depression.

If you notice a loved one suffering, it is my recommendation that she seek help. However, suggesting that she go to therapy may feel invalidating to her, and so I would be gentle and compassionate, encouraging collaboration as part of the healing process.

For example, instead of saying, "Something is wrong with you; you need therapy," I would suggest saying, "Let's put our heads together and see if we can find a way to make things easier on you right now during this time of great transition."

In talking about the darkest parts of postpartum depression, it is important that clinicians and family members recognize the difference between the typical, fleeting scary thoughts that a woman may have and times when a woman believes that she will truly act on those scary thoughts. A woman may avoid her baby, seeking care from others. Women who struggle with postpartum depression often ruminate about the fact that they may actually act on the thoughts involving causing harm to their babies or themselves. If a woman is having suicidal ideations, she may believe that her partner or children would be better off without her. Another sign that a woman is having severe postpartum depression is if she is experiencing a profound sense of hopelessness that things will never improve, that she did irreparable damage to her life or family, and that she will forever be lost in a black hole of despair.

Part III
A HOPEFUL STORY

8

❖ ❖

Support as a Key to Recovery

According to Dr. Wenzel, a social support system is defined as people who provide care, concern, and assistance when needed.

When my husband and I started thinking about having a second child, we were warned that two kids do not require double the work; instead, they require one hundred times the work. From the moment that our family morphed into its square, we realized that, for us, those warnings would not hold true. In fact, having two children, despite all of our difficulties, never even seemed like double the work. The enormous jump from no kids to one kid was much greater than from one to two. As a mother, I was used to living with my heart on the outside of my body. I was used to sleepless nights, heart-searing worry, and beautiful, aching love.

Logistically, things were far easier than we had anticipated. I believe that this is in part due to the fact that we waited three and a half years before having a second child, so that by the time my son was born, my daughter was able to do things like letting the dog in from the yard, going into the fridge for a snack, and taking herself to the bathroom. It is a juggling act at times, but it works. Despite my struggles, I haven't felt overwhelmed by having two kids—unless you count feeling overwhelmed with love. And I mean it.

But having two kids does require some tag teaming. My husband usually oversees my daughter's bedtime. It is a special time that they share. He tells her stories; sometimes they are about his childhood, and sometimes they are about *Star Wars*, and sometimes about princesses who live with the My Little Pony dolls. They sing a certain repertoire of songs, and they snuggle. He rocks her. It is very sweet.

One spring night when Belle was a bit younger, I said that I would come in after stories and songs for a snuggle session with my girl. I crawled into her bed and rested my head on the pillow next to her. I felt peaceful in a way that had been elusive for some time. But I felt it.

I asked her if I could sing a song to her, because all I could hear in my head was the chorus to Edward Sharpe and the Magnetic Zeros song "Home": "Home is wherever I'm with you."

Regardless of what was going on in my brain—all of the chemicals and fears and anxieties with which I was trying to cope—I really wanted, more than anything, to be present for my daughter. I rested my head down beside hers. I told her that she is the most special person I have ever known.

"You are kind. Do you know what *kind* means?" I asked.

"Generous?" She looked at me with her Atlantic Ocean eyes. "At least I think I know what it means!" and we giggled. I told her that she is good. And that she is kind. And that she is smart. And that she is talented. And that she is a great singer (which she took as a cue to sing "Laaaaa" with a perfect vibrato). I told her that she is beautiful. And that she is special. And that she makes everyone around her smile.

She told me that I am special because I show her so much love. Tears filled my eyes.

"If you could have one wish in the whole world, what would it be?" I asked.

"I would wish for a mermaid tail," she said, without pausing to think. "What would your wish be, Mama?"

"I wish that you could be happy every single day of your life," I told her.

"Well, then, that's good, because your wish is going to come true. You always make me happy." And the tears poised in my eyes grew bigger.

We snuggled in the dark silence for a few minutes.

"Mommy?" she asked. "My wish isn't going to come true, is it?"

"Probably not, sweetheart." This was hard for me. I love magic and enchantment, and the last thing that I want to do is to raise a cynic, but I also want to avoid raising a daughter who feels as though she cannot trust me.

"Then I am going to change my wish. I wish that you are happy every single day of your life," she said.

I could hold the tears back no longer.

I know that my daughter will have some sad days, and I wish with all of my might that I could prevent them, but I know that they are inevitable, no matter how many minutes I spend cuddling with and doting on her.

But if she can feel loved every day, then I am doing my job.

"I am going to tell you a secret before I leave," I whispered to her, so quietly that she could barely hear. "You are my heart."

I placed her tiny hand on my chest. "Do you remember how we did that puzzle today and how for a while those pieces were missing? Well, before you, I was like that puzzle. I had pieces missing. And then you came, and you filled up my puzzle and made me whole."

I could barely get out the words. I was "crying happy," as she says.

And she leaned in close to me and put her hand on my cheek and looked into my wet eyes.

"*I* am going to tell *you* a secret now, Mama. I saw Queen Elsa today. And guess what? She had *real* ice powers. But she was *not* wearing nail polish."

And, at that point, all I could do was laugh. We had been through so much in the months prior and so many of the things that had happened to our family would have seemed unbelievable, so who was I to tell her that strange, unexplainable things are anything less than possible?

And so, once again, we resumed our positions in the darkness of her bedroom, locked up like pieces of a perfect puzzle, until she drifted off to sleep. I untangled myself and got out of her bed, quietly, but before leaving I kissed her bow-shaped lips and crouched down to her ear: "Be this happy—this innocent—for the rest of your life, sweet girl. And don't stop believing in mermaid tails."

❖ ❖

A few years after my battle with postpartum depression, while reading the news and checking my social media feeds, I decided to take a quick look at what was going on in the celebrity tabloid world. I saw all of the serious, tragic news stories, but I paused when I started to see Hayden Panettiere's name popping up all over my social media feed.

Ms. Panettiere had, at the time, been a face for postpartum depression advocacy, after coming out with the story of her struggle and sharing her holistic treatment for the affliction. In opening up about her struggle, she said that her postpartum depression had impacted every aspect of her life. And while I felt so grateful for her advocacy, I recognized the pain behind her smile. After all, I knew that look well.

The stories that were being picked up more recently, though, were more "gossip-like," in that they were focused on her relationship. Apparently, she had been spotted and photographed sitting on a stoop and she was *not* wearing her signature, large engagement ring. And, as happens, the Internet started talking: *Her relationship must be over. Or at least in crisis. Is it because of her postpartum depression?*

And I want to say that while it is none of my business, I can understand how her struggle with postpartum depression may (or may not) have affected her marriage. Do I know any of the intimacies or intricacies for sure? No. Have I been there? Yes. Very much so.

Because, and this is something not often addressed, marriage is one of the silent casualties of postpartum depression and, I would venture to say, all major mental health issues. I say this—admit to this—with some serious trepidation, but in an effort to help others I will say that my prenatal and postpartum depression—and the period that has followed—has had an effect on my marriage.

In many ways, it has changed us for the better. It fortified us in ways that I had never thought possible. I have written about this, and I will write more, but first I want to be brutally honest in sharing how it has rocked us, knocked at us, and, at times, divided us.

I am not going to go into every detail, as that would be agonizing, intrusive, and not just my story to tell, but I will say that because it was Kenny who first noticed that something was not right with me in those ten days after the birth of our son, he became the "point person" in our "save the Becca" mission.

When he asked me if I was OK, when he saw "the light going out" in my eyes, he was not really asking literally, but rather rhetorically, I now realize. He knew that I was not OK. He was just doing three things: he was giving me the "reality check" encouraged by the social worker at the hospital, he was expressing his love for me, and he was giving me *permission* to let go. He was saying, without using the words, that I was allowed to admit that I was struggling. I could break down, and he would catch me. Little did he know.

In the months after our son was born, Kenny took over for everyone. He became the world's best husband and "super dad." He watched me fade away, physically and emotionally. He watched my weight wither and my mind go fuzzy. He watched me act out. And through it all, he didn't go anywhere. He was by my side. If he made any movement at all, it was closer to me. He was the most solid of rocks.

And I put all of my weight on him for so long, and when someone who is (albeit physically tiny, but emotionally) extremely heavy leans on a rock, relentlessly, endlessly, that rock, no matter how solid, will start to crack as well.

My husband's story is his own and not mine to share, so I will respect his privacy. But I will say that my illness had an incredible impact on him. He was not the "identified patient"; yet he had to suffer as much as I was, and sometimes probably more. The only thing worse than going through a devastating illness is watching your most cherished loved one go through it, I believe. And for him, it was so, so hard.

But he stayed. Cracks and all.

However, he became more of a caretaker to my sick person as opposed to the loving partner to my own loving partner self. I was not one. I was distant and strange and erratic and not the woman with whom he had fallen in love. He could no longer see me as the strong woman he had once known, because I had lost all of my strength; I was fragile and had physically shrunken away. Kenny had to deal with this while simultaneously taking care of two children, working as our breadwinner at a very busy and important job, and trying to meet his own basic needs.

There is an equation in here somewhere, and it isn't scientific or exact, but it goes something like this:

$$\text{Romantic love} + \text{incredible stress} + \text{illness} + \text{pain} + \text{hurt} = \text{less romantic love}$$

If I am being brutally honest, I will say what I was hinting at above: If this experience showed me anything about my husband, it is that he is *there*. Rather, he is *here*. If I am in hell, he is going to go right down into the depths of hell with me, no matter how scorching it is, and even if his clothing gets burned off and he can't breathe in the smoky, soot-filled air.

But can I please tell you what hell is not? A great place for a date night. Or an ideal spot in which to try to connect.

Hell is hell.

I opened up to my friends about my feelings about the shift in our marriage, and everyone cheered us on. "Look at how much you guys have endured. You are the most *amazing* couple," they would say.

But one conversation stuck with me more than any other. Interestingly enough, this conversation was with a male friend, who has independent relationships with both Kenny and me, and he and I were talking very candidly about love, life, and marriage—how all of these things are so wonderful but also so hard. With some reservations, but a surge of bravery,

I opened up to my friend about the fact that while my husband and I have so many strengths, like an incredible friendship and similar interests and coinciding values, I sometimes wonder about our passion. Are we an amazing family together or are we fiery lovers? The former seemed obvious; the latter, less so.

And my friend looked at me and said something that I did not expect.

"It depends on how you define passion. I am not sure how you two define it, but to me, I know that Kenny just let you nap while he went into your closet and packed up your *entire* collection of clothing, put all of your shoes into trash bags, and took care of your things. To me, that shows a level of deep love. And maybe *that* is passion."

My friend was right. Just like so many other things that Kenny had done for me since the fall of 2013, he took care of me in a small but huge way. I had been tired and taken a rest, and I did not ask him to pack up my closet for me. It most certainly was not fun. But he did it. He did not ask for thanks or credit. He just did it. He did something to make my life easier because he loves me, and that is what he does.

Is that the passion that is shown in movies and written about in romance novels? Not even close.

But is it love? Absolutely.

When I think about Hayden Panettiere and her husband, I can only imagine the struggles that they must have endured during her darkest days. Having a baby is hard enough, and being a celebrity adds an increased amount of scrutiny and pressure. And so was he her rock during this time? I have no idea. And is that why she was not wearing her six-carat diamond while reading on a stoop? I don't know the answer to that, either. Will she and her husband continue to post family pictures proclaiming their love and happiness and then later announce their split? Only time will tell.

But I will tell you that postpartum depression is insidious in nature, because it is extreme devastation, packaged along with an incredibly cute baby, whom you're supposed to love and adore. And feel lucky to have. And do you know what is worse than feeling deep depression? Feeling deep depression when the world tells you that you are supposed to be happier than ever. Family photos from that time so often belie the realities: that sleepless nights cause couples to bicker with exhaustion and newborns take up so much time that there is little time to foster a romantic relationship.

I wish Hayden the best. If her marriage is fine and has withstood this arduous test, then I am thrilled for her. If it could not, there is no shame in that, and I hope that they find peace, together or apart. It is hard to be sick, both for the sufferer and for her support system. Mental health issues can be even trickier, as they are diseases that cannot be seen on the outside or measured with bloodwork or a CT scan.

I am not here to say that prenatal or postpartum depression causes all affected marriages to get weaker or stronger. But I do believe that prenatal and postpartum distress do impact everyone involved in the situation, because it did for me. I lost some friends and found incredible closeness with others; I have leaned on my family in ways that I had never thought possible. My marriage has changed—it has grown. Kenny and I are closer than ever, for better or for worse, in sickness and in health.

It is important, though, to recognize a hard truth: once you go to hell with someone, it is impossible to forget the trip as if it never happened. Even when you reemerge, your clothes will likely still have that smoky smell, you may have bandages from third-degree burns, and, well . . . you've just been to hell.

So you find a new path. And that path doesn't always lead to the same place that you were before, and it does not always lead people back to each other. But the best you can do is to get on that path and start walking. Hand in hand, or on your own two feet or whatever is best for you and your family. For Kenny and me, it has meant working with a therapist, putting in hard work and strengthening our bond in new and different ways. It has meant connecting on all levels. It has meant being honest about the hardest of truths, and also letting go of the things that no longer serve us.

All I can tell you is that my husband and I are both survivors. I was the one to give birth and to experience the acute symptoms of my affliction, but he was right there with me, a solid but sometimes cracking rock. And I am eternally grateful for all that he has given and all that he has done.

Marriage is complicated and can be difficult in the best of circumstances.

Whenever I remember to do so, I stop him and I say, "Thank you, Kenny. Thank you for being my rock. If I had to be in hell, there is no one else with whom I would have rather had by my side." Because the truth is that when we were down there, down at the very bottom, where the worst, scariest things are kept, it was Kenny who gave me his last remaining shreds of clothing—anything that had not been burned off. He put the cloth around my shoulders, wrapped me up, and made sure that I was protected from the fire, as flames licked his own exposed body.

He is an amazing human being. He put my shoes in trash bags. I could even say that he *rocked* it.

And the world should know.

FROM DR. WENZEL

A positive social support system is crucial for a woman who is recovering from any form of perinatal distress. Support can come in many forms, including a woman's spouse or partner, friends, children, therapist, family members, doctors, doulas, lactation consultants, support groups, online forums, and psychopharmacologists.

Psychologists have identified several types of support that can be provided by members of one's social support network. They are as follows:

Emotional support is defined as the support experienced when a woman has a person or people who are *truly* there for her, providing her with warmth, care, and validation.

Informational support is defined as factual advice or resources that a woman can use in times of need. Rebecca's blog is an example of informational support, as she gives her readers guidance by putting a name to their feelings and referring them to resources for different types of help. In fact, mommyeverafter.com is a great example of the way in which emotional support and informational support can work hand in hand, as Rebecca's online community for women is a hub for emotional support while also giving readers the usable advice of informational support.

Tangible support is the actual help that a person can provide to a mother or family. Practical examples of tangible support include a person who stays overnight to get up with the baby so that the mom can sleep, a person who changes diapers, or a person who can go shopping for the woman and family so that these burdens are lifted.

A positive support system is a most critical part of a woman's recovery. That said, despite good intentions, it is possible that a woman will be faced with negative social support, defined as support that is experienced as unhelpful or unwanted. It is important to note that oftentimes such support is well intentioned; however, in actuality, it is experienced as annoying, disruptive, or even painful.

This is a delicate tightrope on which to walk. Many people, especially family members, offer "help" in the form of unsolicited advice, which can trigger negative emotions rather than being helpful. For example, there is the "When I was pregnant . . ." generation, who have very strong ideas about how things should be: "When I was pregnant I used to smoke cigarettes and eat deli meat." Not only is this antiquated advice unsupportive, but it can also be agitating. Effective communication is crucial in setting boundaries and keeping peace for everyone, especially for the woman. It is a dance.

One tool that people can use to set boundaries and provide healing is the *positive-negative-positive sandwich*. People who use this tool first start with saying something positive or encouraging to another, then follow with something that has the potential to be perceived by the other as negative (e.g., making a request, setting a boundary, providing criticism), and subsequently follow with another positive or encouraging statement. Successful implementation of this tool often results in the person on the receiving end of the communication being more receptive to the negative message that the individual is attempting to communicate. If a new mother has intrusive people in her life who give unsolicited advice, giving them criticism has the potential to breed defensiveness and tension. This scenario could lead to a power struggle, the last thing that anyone, especially a new mother, needs.

Take, for example, a situation in which a new mother's mother-in-law is not caring for the infant in a way that is consistent with the new mother's wishes, placing the infant on his stomach for a nap. Instead of confrontation, the interaction could be structured as follows:

1. The new mother could express gratitude for the aid and expertise of her "supporter" (e.g., "Thank you so much for all of your help and for offering to do the baby's nap; that is so kind of you").
2. Then she could use the opportunity to express her wishes to her mother-in-law in a clear and kind way (e.g., "I know that this is different from how you did things when you had children, but now babies are to be placed to sleep on their backs, as it has been shown to lower the risk for SIDS; I learned all about this in my classes leading up to childbirth").
3. Then she could follow with a statement about how helpful it is to be learning together (e.g., "Isn't it interesting how things change over the years? Again, thank you for offering to do nap time and for now making sure that the baby is always on her back; I know this must feel so different, so I guess we are all learning together").

Being able to provide feedback in a way that a family member can hear is difficult, yet vital, as it serves to validate the help that this person *is* providing.

1. I am so grateful that you are here to help our family. I look forward to learning together.
2. Thank you for allowing me to rest, changing the diapers, and running to the store for me. I am so grateful.

Another effective communication skill is the *broken record technique*, in which a person repeats the same request or expresses the same opinion each time she is met with opposition. In other words, the person repeats the main message much like a vinyl record that has a scratch on it, rather than being derailed by resistance from the other person. The use of this tool requires a new mother to be clear about her wants and needs. When a member of the negative support system tries to talk about his or her own experience, the mother responds by pulling the conversation back to the main point, avoiding excessive detail or dragging in past history. It is important to use a calm, even voice when using the broken record technique, as well as to apply it consistently. The goal is to be assertive (i.e., firm but respectful of others) rather than aggressive.

I encourage women to be mindful of their personal preferences for communication and interactions with others during pregnancy and to use knowledge of those preferences to guide the selections of professionals who will provide them support. For example, when I had my daughter, I was eager for specific guidance and information. I wanted someone to tell me what to do and how to do it. Despite my clinical knowledge, I did not feel confident in taking care of a newborn, so I was happy to get hands-on, concrete advice. By contrast, after her deliveries, Rebecca was emotional and sensitive and wanted a "warm and fuzzy" postpartum doula who would provide praise and comfort. Having professionals in place whose style matches a new mother's personal style has the potential to ease the transition to parenthood.

Negative social support can seem overwhelming, and it is tempting to shut out the sources of such stress. As hard as it is, new mothers should remember that this is a time of great upheaval and transition, and they might later regret concluding that a relationship is not salvageable even if the support they are receiving from that individual at the time is not helpful.

Instead of dwelling on negative support, I suggest that a woman simply take a step back and devote the most time possible to her positive supporters. She need not feel shamed or guilted into spending time with the person or people who are causing her stress; instead, she can direct her energy and focus on the supporters who *do* promote positivity, confidence, and security. It is important to remember that everyone makes judgments based on their own frame of reference, so it is very possible that comments that are experienced by the new mother as unhelpful were made with the best of intentions.

In all, during the perinatal period, a woman needs to do whatever it takes to survive. She must grant herself permission to take care of *herself*. Childbirth changes things for everyone. Women have many expectations, and there will, inevitably, be moments of disappointment. This is normal. The time after welcoming a baby is so charged, and carries so much meaning, that the best thing that a woman can do to arm herself for success is to go into the experience as prepared as possible. By using effective communication and by taking some of the pressure off of herself by adjusting expectations, a woman should be better equipped to handle the inevitably emotional postpartum period.

9

❖ ❖

Together, Ever After

I started writing my blog, *Mommy, Ever After*, in June 2010, when Belle was just two months old. I originally looked at the site as my online baby book and would post my past pregnancy stories, funny parenthood anecdotes, and revelations about how motherhood, while enchanting, can also be hard, scary, lonely, boring, and, most certainly, unpredictable.

After my anxiety-filled pregnancy and Beau's birth in 2013, I came out with my story of postpartum depression in a post titled "The Hardest Post I've Ever Written." This piece turned my little blog into an international platform from which I could help other women, comfort their family members and caregivers, and create a private online support group for women across the country.

In this chapter, you will read the stories of five women, each of whom shares their struggles with perinatal distress. The parallels between their stories and my story are staggering. These stories are brutal accounts of prenatal anxiety and sadness, postpartum depression, and the overwhelming sense of shame associated with these afflictions. There is also a call to action. Each woman independently sought help and, without any guidance, wrote to implore readers to do the same.

I write to help other women and their families so that they do not have to suffer like I did—like my family did. If this chapter shows nothing else, it is an illustration that none of us are alone. These problems are universal and pervasive and real. And instead of feeling isolated, we can feel together. Ever after.

AMIE, THIRTY-FOUR YEARS OLD

Tears start to stream down my face as I begin to write about my experience with postpartum anxiety and depletion after my second baby girl, Juliet. It is a mix of happy tears and tears of hardship as I remember my oys and joys of second-time-around mommyhood. Sharing my story feels like something I both need and want to do. Throughout my journey to recovery, I've felt shame and guilt, and the inevitable "but why me?" I have shared my woes with certain people, but many people don't know this about me. I am only beginning to feel the bravery in opening up about this and have now come to understand that displaying my weakness feels more like a strength.

This postpartum depression plague feels like one of the most difficult things to explain. In a way, I'm at a loss for words. However, I'm not going to allow sharing my story to defeat me. I'll go back and remember walking through those muddy waters. The only thing I can do is tell my view, my perspective, my experience, my truth.

I wonder if after people who know me, knew me, will always look at me in a different way. In a more negative light. She could not hack it. Or there's something wrong with her. I do care what other people think. There isn't a role on earth, an experience, I would rather have than motherhood. It is my jam. I love my two little girls to bits and pieces. Their happiness is my happiness. I'm honored to call them mine.

Being a mother is both the hardest and the most rewarding thing I believe I will ever do in my life. It is a dream come true for me, and I so enjoy my girls. And I know that they know it. I stop during the day, all the time, to give them kisses and snuggles. We have giggle fits and dance parties, and I tell them I love them more times than I can count. I am silly with them, so much so that I think that they think that I am their littermate, their equal. I have days when I feel like I'm floating on air, and, to be honest, most of those days entail a few hours away from them, to recharge, exercise, write, read, whatever I need. And when I'm with them on those days it sometimes feels like magic. I think this is the best. I'm so lucky. I will never need time away again. I have got it all figured out. What was all that whining from before? But from this experience I've learned the importance of self-care, and not to take it for granted. While I'm loving motherhood, I am also just trying to get through the day. It's a hard job *without* a blanket of personal anxiety having severely suffocated me.

After the birth of my first daughter I was so amazingly happy and joyful. I have had a good amount of experience with childcare over the years, so I did not have much of a learning curve. The only hump that I had to get over was from those two new heaping humps on my chest: nursing. My milk supply was huge. So much so that I could have probably fed triplets, but I was in so much pain each and every time I nursed that it felt like needles, and I wondered when that pain would go away. After a couple of months, I could finally breastfeed my baby without any trouble. My stubbornness and stick-to-itiveness paid off. I cherished each day with Stella, not ever wanting another day to pass. That said, I also felt exhausted and complained about how trying it could be. But all in all I was happy. My dreams had come true. I had a wonderful family. My husband and I wanted to have children close in age, and thought, "Why wait?" So I got pregnant again a few months after Stella's first birthday.

I had a normalish pregnancy the second time around. But something was not the same. A big something. I was not able to relax and rest and enjoy many pregnant moments like I did with my first pregnancy. I felt pretty tired and suffered from morning sickness for the first several months of my pregnancy. I got plenty of sleep at night, giving myself a bedtime of approximately nine in the evening, and tried to nap when Stella napped. I gained about forty-five pounds again, about the same as with Stella. There were more external stress factors than when I was pregnant with my first child, but my mood was generally fine.

My water broke a few weeks before my due date, on April Fool's Day. Unlike with Stella, where it felt like gallons of water endlessly coming out of me, it was just a little bit of fluid. And I thought, "Is this it?" It was confusing, and unsettling, but after my husband and I went to the hospital, the nurse ran some tests and I learned that, yes, my water did indeed break. I opted to get induced because I did not want to roam the hospital halls for seventy-two hours, and so I endured the contractions, bedridden, with my hubby by my side. We did not know the sex of the baby that we were having, but since I felt so different this laboring time around, I felt it must be a boy. I started to become convinced of it during my labor.

Many painful, long hours passed slowly, and, finally, it was time to push. Game time. This delivery process brought me all the magic and awe that I had with my first. After only a couple of pushes, Juliet came out of my womb and into the world. It was a total surprise to us that she was a girl. And I was over the moon for her. John and I both were. We fell madly in love with this lovely little girl. We decided to name her Juliet Audrey, because that means youthful and lovely.

I had a nice, uneventful stay in the hospital. As most dads' messages usually say, we were "doing well. Happy and healthy." That was us.

With this sweet little one, my second baby girl, my milk supply came in right away, and nursing couldn't have been easier this time around. I remember feeling like I was on cloud nine. It was the most wonderful feeling, a euphoria that I cannot even explain. Yes, I was indeed exhausted, but I was also so incredibly happy.

When we got home after the hospital, I was doing well, by my standards. I felt amazing and like I could do anything. In a way, I felt like I was on a high. For weeks, I had family come and go to help us with the new baby and our big transition. Well taken care of with my company, I pushed through all of the sleeplessness and round-the-clock nursing with much more ease than I ever had with my first child. I didn't have any overriding concern for Juliet's well-being. She gained weight beautifully and, as a baby, was "killing it" in all departments.

When the visitors began to dwindle, I started to take care of mostly everything regarding the girls. John certainly pitched in when he was home and is an incredible father to our girls. I couldn't ask for anyone better to help raise our precious babies.

And then it got hard.

After about a month, I noticed a change starting to occur within myself. I felt irritable more often than not, overwhelmed, anxious, moody, lonely, sad, and, even more than that, depressed. In the beginning, these feelings came in waves. Waves I could control with routine and discipline. My brain felt different, like the wiring wasn't working properly. It was as if my brain was a record player. Skip. Skip and scratch. My thoughts would scramble together, and I would wait for the next stopping point. I do not mean to describe the so-called normal times of brain-drain after having a new baby; this was not a sleepless baby fog, but something that felt a million times worse. If I knew that I would be seeing other people, and I knew that I would have to be social, I would have to strain very hard to focus. Socializing felt hard for me, but I imagine that if you were on the outside looking in, it wasn't noticeable. That is the problem sometimes with mental illnesses: others can't see the elephant in the room that you feel. It is crushing, yet invisible to the world.

I should back up and be completely honest: I am naturally more of an introvert than an extrovert. In the past, even before children, socializing gave me some anxiety. However, this time it felt as if a magnifying glass was being held up to all of my anxiety. As if, instead of a small part of my body holding a little anxiety, my entire self—my entire being—were consumed with it. And the anxiety did not just stop with socializing. Absolutely everything about me gave me anxiety. It was mentally crippling. At times, it felt like I was dying.

Just like with Stella, the pounds began to melt off of me. I wasn't doing much, aside from breastfeeding, to help that process along. My healthy little chunker took a lot out of me. I ate all the time, tried to choose healthy things, but didn't start any crazy exercise routine. I tried to take care of myself, but my efforts felt more like failures.

When the months started blending together, I wasn't quite sure how I could hold it together anymore. On several different occasions, when both children were napping and I finally had alone time, I would hit a breaking point and find myself in tears. I made phone calls to the nurses at my OBGYN's practice. I told them about my symptoms, and they let me know that they could prescribe me medication. Over the phone. Just like that. I wasn't OK with that answer. I didn't need any medicine after my first child. I never needed any medication before. I was scared and, most of all, stubborn about taking something. But each time I called, I felt my symptoms getting worse and worse.

I had never felt this kind of agony before, and with the huge responsibility of caring for two young children, practically around the clock, I did not even know where to begin to take care of myself or seek treatment. I didn't know what I had or what was taking over me. I found it difficult to open up to people about how I was feeling. And when I began to, I felt I was met with more dismissive comments like "Yup, it is hard with two kids." I knew it was hard, but there was something going on with me that wasn't right. I would often have to go into (what I would refer to as) robot mode; it felt like I had to turn on, charge up, and activate in order take care of them. I should note something that I find interesting about my anxiety: I did not feel very anxious about my children, nor did I obsess over every single thing. I continued to put my all into caring for them, and they were really doing quite well.

Externally, from what I believe, my condition would have been very hard to notice. Though, on the inside, I felt like I was carrying around the heaviest weights within me. While I enjoyed spending time with my children, everything was beginning to feel like so much of a chore, and I was missing out on any of the enjoyment. Though I tried, and I did so with all of the might that I could muster, I could not get myself back. I could not even recognize myself.

I am a stay-at-home mom, so I work—yes, work—around the clock. That meant that I could not possibly find the time to figure out what I needed. My husband felt like I was being more bitchy, resentful, and moody when I spoke about it to him. He was confused about me, and he had a lot on his plate to deal with on his own. "Wasn't this what you wanted?" he asked.

"You have what you always wanted," I imagined him thinking.

Finding help for myself was not an easy task. First, I had to admit defeat in a way and hand myself over to a greater power. And having been so strongly in mom mode, my priority was no longer caring for myself but caring for my children. So it seemed backward for me to think about myself first: the old, but so aptly put, adage about putting that oxygen mask on myself first. I wasn't very familiar with seeking psychological treatment and felt like finding someone who took my insurance was an insurmountable task.

I also took the Edinburgh test at my six-week checkup at the OBGYN's office. The memory is now a blur and I don't remember filling out that test; I think that I must have been in a fog. That, combined with being a mom who really wanted to ace motherhood and admit nothing was wrong, caused me to fudge the answers. Yes, I cheated on the "Are you OK?" exam. I wanted so badly to pretend I was really doing all right. I didn't want to spark the discussion with my nurses or doctors in person. And I am pretty sure that my children were with me at the appointment, and so it was impossible for me to fathom getting into any meaningful conversation. At home, I often scored myself, honestly, on the Edinburgh Postnatal Depression Scale, and the numbers showed clearly that I was, in fact, suffering from postpartum depression. I knew it, even if no one else knew the depths of my struggle.

For me it was more of a culminating experience leading to a perfect storm that I had to recover from and, if I am being honest, am still recovering from. And this perfect storm happened, ironically, on a family vacation.

While on our annual family trip to the beach, with my extended family, all my loved ones, I really felt worse than ever before. Juliet was four months old. Too many months had gone by without any help, and deep down I knew it. I was exclusively nursing Juliet, her sleep schedule was not consistent, and I felt as if I had a really low energy supply. I felt depleted, annoyed, and sad. I could cry incredibly easily, about anything, and I knew that it wasn't a normal feeling. I knew how wrong I felt, that nothing about how I felt seemed OK anymore, but it was really the last place I wanted to talk to anyone about it. I felt if asked "How are you?" that I would simply crumble and start a long, uncontrollable sob story. So I easily hid behind my cute girls and their adorable outfits, and I myself put on a bit more makeup, dressed up, and hid in plain sight. I went into stealth mode, hiding in the bathroom, finally getting on the phone with some psychologists, trying to reach out to someone who could help me. I managed to make an appointment the week I got back, and I found some peace in that.

My husband had to get back to work midweek, so I stayed at the beach with my family in Rhode Island. I drove the five hours home on Saturday morning, and I did so while I was in a bad way. I drove with my mom in the passenger seat next to me, and my two little cuties in the back, and any sad song that played on the radio would make me cry. I confided in my mom that I really wasn't doing well at all. I told her about my appointment and told her to remind me that when I got home and my routine could start again, that I was really not OK and that it would be extremely important for me to seek help. With about an hour left of the ride, my mom had to get out of our car and into my brother's car, at a rest stop, since they were both going home together.

As I drove I could feel myself breaking, the cracks exposed, the pain that I had been suppressing beginning to pour out, and about a half hour away from home, while going over a bridge, I could feel my body shutting down. I was actually, in every way I can explain, shutting down. I was in full-on panic mode, and I no longer felt I had any control over the wheel or any semblance of balance. I am certain that a higher power got me to the side of the road, right before a toll booth, and I managed to flag someone down. I was having a full-fledged panic attack and I thought that I was dying. While going over the bridge, I called John, and I tried to communicate to him where we were, so he could come get us, but all I could do was mutter the numbers to the exit I saw ahead. So when I flagged a lady down who worked at the toll booth, I had her talk to my husband to tell him where I was. I think I kept uttering something about postpartum depression and needing water.

Luckily, nobody got hurt. There was no accident. On the outside, I was safe and everything was fine. Even the girls in the back were awake and being complete angels during this traumatic episode.

Inside of my body was a different story. My storm had hit a record high and I was not doing well. The storm had taken over, and the bad, sad, and scary emotions were swirling like a cyclone. A fire ambulance came; people came to check my pulse. I like to play by the rules. I do not like to cause a scene, and I was causing a big scene.

I began feeling really paranoid and scared. John finally arrived, got us, and drove us home. When I got home I thought that I would just lie down in bed, take a nap, and that magically everything would be better. Before my nap, I showered, and yet, despite my hopes, I could not relax. I was amped up, buzzing, freaked out, and I began to really think that I was dying. I had a bathroom floor moment, where I lay there, thinking, "This is it. I must be having a heart attack and dying." I had my husband call 911. An ambulance came and took me to the hospital.

I thought I would be admitted to a psychiatric ward of a hospital and that my girls would be taken away from me. I really had no clue about postpartum depression, and I did not realize that finally giving over to it, saying that I needed help, asking for assistance, would help me finally begin to get better, and not worse.

In the emergency room I was given Ativan, an antianxiety medicine, for panic disorders. It did not help much to ward off any anxiety or panic. Without feeling much better, or any better, for that matter, John got me from the hospital and took me home. My parents got our daughters from us so that John could help me to rest. In the back of my mind, in some disturbed part, I still thought that my children might be taken away from me. That since I showed my weakness, I would be punished, and that I would only continue to get worse. I had no idea what was taking over me, but it was heavy and powerful and palpable and pervasive. I remember John putting me to bed, and I told him to please watch over me to make sure I was still breathing since I thought my heart was going to stop beating any moment.

Giving over to the fact that, yes, I was struggling—admitting to having postpartum depression—was so internally difficult for me. It still is. But it helped me begin my road to recovery.

Since I felt like my head was not on straight, I began to lose some of my confidence in being a mom. I needed backup. We initially had to hire a full-time nanny, so that I could take care of myself and the children properly. Initially, I hated that idea. I did not in any way want someone coming in and taking over. I thought my bond with my girls would weaken with help, but I was so wrong. It was the best thing I could have done for myself and my family, and it was temporary. It allowed me to get off of the hamster wheel of anxiety and despair, as it allowed me to take breaks, to pursue hobbies, to exercise, to go to therapy, to have one-on-one time with each child. I could, finally, put my shoulders down a bit and breathe more easily for a while. I was extremely worried about money, the financial strains that I had, and would, put on us while getting better, but I also knew it was the only way.

That next week I had an appointment at my OBGYN's office. I met with a nurse who shared that she had also experienced postpartum depression. She initially checked my blood pressure, and my anxiety reached a new level; I thought that she was going to say that I was doing horribly and that she had never seen blood pressure so low or high in all of her time as a nurse. It seemed all roads in my mind kept leading to the fact that I was dying. I *believed* this. Yet, in reality, my blood pressure was perfect; just the thoughts in my head and the anxiety in my system were not. We talked about what I could do to feel better, and talked about the possibility of me taking medication, like an antidepressant for relief. She also ordered tests to check for anemia and thyroid dysfunction.

My blood lab results came back normal. It was almost a bit disappointing because I'd rather pinpoint the pain than keep searching for the reason I felt so bad. Finally, a few days after this visit, I felt I couldn't hold on any longer on my own, and I opted to take the medication that was prescribed to me. It was a low dose of Zoloft that I learned worked for many women who didn't feel quite right in their postpartum days.

Apparently, you can still breastfeed on this medication. I did not want to give up nursing, but I also thought that I was being too stubborn to say that I was going to continue to solely nurse. We introduced formula, and it felt good to give my body a little break and open up another option.

I also began running again, which helped a bit, because exercise helps release those wonderful endorphins, but it did not help enough. It took a while for the medicine to sink in and work properly. I had to deal with many side effects. The first and worst one was suicidal thoughts. Luckily, I only dealt with that for one afternoon, but it was the worst mental pain I ever felt. I immediately called my family and had them come and help: get me and stay with me. I knew the medicine was learning how to work with my brain, and after a few days, it did help calm my nerves, settle some anxieties, but it also numbed me. I could not cry, even if I wanted to. I was taking a low dose and, after a few months, decided to break the pill in half, and I liked this dose best.

By December I had been taking this medicine for about four months, and I was ready to be done, so on Christmas Day, I stopped taking it. I felt good going into the new year with a New Year's resolution of no more medicine and a clean bill of health. I can remember on New Year's Eve not feeling very good but trying to forge on anyway. At dinner with John, I began to slur my words and it was hard for me to formulate a sentence. And we realized it was not time yet, and it was silly for me to put unnecessary pressures like that on myself or give myself an unreasonable timeline. But I cried, because I wanted to be over all of this already.

At the beginning of my treatment process, a main part of my personal wellness plan was seeing a psychologist at first a couple times a week, then once a week, and finally to eliminate regularly scheduled sessions. Getting involved in wonderful moms groups helped me look at therapy in a whole new wonderful light.

While I almost hit rock bottom, I knew deep down there was only one way to go, and that was up. I needed constant reassurance that I was going to be OK. Those words felt good to me to hear, even though I felt anything but that was the truth. My path was confusing and murky, but I knew I needed to put my mental health at the forefront. Most of it was dealing with a whole lot of anxiety. My anxiety was so bad that I felt like I was going to have a panic attack at times. I felt like it would slowly trickle in and fill me up. Through therapy and taking better care of myself, I learned coping mechanisms. Sometimes all of the tricks up my sleeve wouldn't work, and only time was the cure. Hoping the next day would be easier. I felt I had a very sensitive nervous system and it would get shot more often than not. This is not something to be taken lightly, and I feel that without treatment it continues to get worse and worse.

Having breaks from my children at first made me feel horribly guilty, but I began to see the need to recharge as a healthy thing. I am so grateful for my soul searching, for weeding my mental garden, planting positive seeds, and feeling really great. Worthy. It felt for a long time like I was fighting a losing battle. Climbing uphill I was not feeling a natural state of well-being. I felt bad. It helped me pivot in a new direction because I learned what wasn't working, like comparing myself to others. Caring what people think of me. Thinking I should be doing more than what I was and am doing.

I have learned that perinatal distress is not something that just goes away after taking a pill, getting a babysitter, or getting a good night's sleep. It is an ongoing process and a strong crush to the ego, but I am in a wonderful place right now. That said, this newfound peace still does not mean there are not days that I wake up feeling a bit of that weight creeping in again, feeling my thoughts getting scrambled again, wishing I could lie in bed an extra hour or two and not respond to anything going on around me.

Now, I try to count my blessings more. I have an appreciation journal on my bedside table that reads, "Love the life you live. Live the life you love." A quote from Bob Marley. I try to take it easier on myself. This is not something you can ace after a week, or even a year. It is sensitive, close to home, and can be scary.

As a mom dealing with postpartum issues, I really wanted to connect with others who faced this terrible affliction. I found so much comfort in reading *Mommy, Ever After* and every one of Rebecca's blog posts, and I reached out to her. Quickly, she became a friend of mine, a confidant. No matter what, she told me, "you do you." Wise words. Take care of yourself first every day, whatever that healthy and happy looks like to you. Everyone else around you will reap the rewards of your well-being. That's my journey now. Now, I have a new story. And now I have hope.

ERICA, FORTY-FOUR YEARS OLD

The baby was crying. She wouldn't stop. I had to make her stop. I grabbed her off the bed and threw her on the floor. And she was finally quiet. Except she was not. She was still on the bed, crying. I grabbed her and threw her on the floor again. And again. This scene played over and over in my mind until I fell to the ground myself, sobbing, shaking.

I had been crying for five months. I cried while I did the laundry; I cried while I sat in my office working. I told my friends and family that I thought something was wrong with me. "No," they said. "You are the strongest person we know. You can handle anything, so you will handle whatever this is." Every weekday morning, I drove over the bridge between my home and my job and pictured myself driving off the edge into the river below. I imagined my car sinking into the water. I couldn't figure out why this was happening. I didn't want to die. I definitely wasn't suicidal. Maybe I wanted things to stop, or at least slow down, but not by killing myself. I needed to figure this out and fix it. I was strong, the strongest person my friends knew, so I could fix this, right?

I dreaded driving to work in the morning, and then I spent the day dreading the ride home. I knew that bridge was waiting for me, tempting me. As I drove across each day, I felt my body trying to react. My hands clenched on the steering wheel, my brain signaling my arms to turn the wheel, while something inside me prevented this movement and kept me straight on the path to the other side of the river. I never felt like I was actually going to drive off the road, but part of me wanted to. And yet I didn't want to die. How could I want to engage in a suicidal act but not be suicidal? I was confused and frustrated that I couldn't figure this out and make it stop.

This went on for five long months. I chatted with coworkers and neighbors and answered with a smile when they asked about the baby. Everyone remarked on my happy glow of motherhood. I was pretty sure that was just oily skin from not showering more than once a week, if that, but I smiled and said, "Thank you," like a robot programed to respond. Each time I opened up to someone and confided that I was crying all the time and didn't feel right, I got the same reply: I was strong and fine.

For five months I was hanging on by a thread. And then, in a moment, that thread snapped. I was in my bedroom, holding the baby. I don't recall anything out of the ordinary, recognizing that "ordinary" at that point was severe sleep deprivation and overwhelming stress. But there is nothing that I can remember as a "last straw," no obvious triggering event. Rather, I suddenly felt unsafe. I was terrified. I put the baby on the bed, as close to the center as possible, so she wouldn't roll off the edge. She started to cry when I put her down. I needed to think. I needed her to stop crying, so I could think. I was in a panic. Something was happening, and I didn't know what or why. I looked at the baby and imagined picking her up and throwing her on the floor. I imagined it over and over again, all the while horrified that my mind was envisioning hurting my child, the child I loved more than anything in the world. I had to make it stop. I wasn't this kind of person. I wasn't a mother who would hurt her baby or even think of hurting her baby, ever. I was sobbing uncontrollably, and I fell to the floor, a broken heap of scared and lonely and helpless. My mind raced, searching for answers. I remembered a handout I was given by the social worker in the maternity ward. It was on blue paper. I needed to find that blue paper. I dug through a stack of paperwork to find the discharge folder from the hospital. Blue paper, blue paper. I tore the papers out of the folder, letting them scatter on the floor. Blue! I saw blue! I grabbed the blue paper. It was the handout I remembered, describing signs of postpartum depression. It said if I had any of the following symptoms, I should call my obstetrician. I had all the symptoms.

I called the number I knew by heart. I was near hysterics. When the receptionist answered, I managed to choke out my name and that I needed to speak to my doctor. For the first time in my twenty years as a patient at this practice, someone went and got the doctor instead of telling me that he would call me back when he could. I can only imagine how desperate I sounded.

My doctor, whom I adored, despite his reputation for being "cold," got on the phone within seconds and asked me what was going on. I was crying so hard that I could barely breathe, let alone speak. I said, "Something is wrong with me. I can't stop crying. Something is wrong. Something is wrong. I need help." And he calmly told me that it would be OK, that it sounded like I was suffering from postpartum depression. He said he was going to call in a prescription for me and I needed to find a way to pick it up or to have someone else pick it up for me if I couldn't safely get myself to the pharmacy. He said that unfortunately it often took up to two weeks for the medication to take effect and we would need to figure out the best next steps. And in that moment, I felt like someone had pulled me back up to the top of the cliff I was dangling from. Someone finally listened to me and helped me. And I felt like maybe things might really be OK.

I remember my doctor asking at the end of the call, "Why did you wait so long to call me?" I told him that I kept telling everyone that something was wrong and I needed help and they told me I didn't. I was in a terrible situation at work, and my friends and coworkers kept reminding me that my boss made lots of people cry in their offices, so this was not a symptom of anything other than working for my boss. And my doctor replied, in his matter-of-fact tone, "Erica, it's never normal to cry for ten hours a day." And I explained, "But you've never met my boss!" And then I burst into laughter, though I was still sobbing. We both laughed, and he told me to start taking the medication immediately. It was the first time in five months that I had felt even a tiny shred of hope, and my entire being was flooded with a sense of relief.

To this day, I remind myself how lucky I was. I have a long history of medical issues, including unusual reactions to medications, and yet I was in the small, yet fortunate, minority who feel the effects of the antidepressant almost immediately. It didn't take two weeks, as the doctor had feared, but rather two days. And that bit of good medical fortune kept me from a path that would surely have been devastating. Over the course of the next few weeks, I saw a number of healthcare professionals, all of whom commented that I had escaped a true crisis by reacting so quickly to the antidepressants. Several told me flat out that if it had taken even one more day for the medication to take effect, it's very likely that I would have had postpartum psychosis. I shudder to think what that progression from depression to psychosis might have meant for my baby and for me, and I remain grateful that I will never know the answer. As it was, my journey was plenty difficult.

My obstetrician sent me to a psychologist who specialized in postpartum mental health issues, and that made me feel even more anxious and stressed. The first step was increasing my antidepressant dose, which turned out to be ill advised. The dose was too high, and I felt completely detached. I didn't feel anxious or depressed, because I didn't feel anything. It was as if I were outside my body, watching myself from a distance. I called my obstetrician and described how I was feeling. He intervened and had the dose lowered, but from that point on, I was nervous about changing my dose.

The facility where I received mental health treatment did not accept insurance, so I was spending more money than I could comfortably afford to on therapy sessions. I didn't hesitate to do this, because I recognized that getting help for myself was critical to my future health and my ability to care for my child. This money, though, was not well spent. My sessions were more damaging than helpful. In fact, they weren't at all helpful. I was taking both time and money that I couldn't afford to sit for an hour and receive useless advice (like telling me to make friends with women who had similar-age babies, so I could trade babysitting with them). This elevated my stress levels dramatically. One day, I patiently explained that I was over forty, did not have any family in the area, worked full-time (at least eighty hours a week) in a single-income household, and had several chronic illnesses that I needed to manage. And that this made it difficult to utilize suggestions to "go out and join playgroups" or "have your mom come and help out" or "quit your job." I said that I was trying to find realistic solutions to reduce my stress levels, and that I was willing to think outside the box and to have my assumptions challenged, but I needed real options. And the mental health professional listened to me, and started to cry, and pronounced, "Your life is so hard! And sad!" And that was my last appointment.

There were no easy answers or quick fixes. The antidepressants made life bearable, but I still couldn't drive over bridges without my mind playing tricks on me. I learned that this was called having "scary thoughts," which made me angry. I felt like a child being told that I was worried about monsters under my bed. I felt only marginally better when I learned that it is also called "suicidal ideation." I wanted a clinical term that accurately captured the experience, and I was angry that there was none. I was angry with myself that I felt ashamed by these thoughts and visions and even by the diagnosis of postpartum depression. I felt weak, like a failure. I couldn't hold it together because I had one baby, and a pretty easy baby at that. I had a running dialogue in my head, where I reminded myself that I hadn't slept more than two consecutive hours since the time I became pregnant and that severe sleep deprivation in itself can cause all sorts of effects on the brain and the body. And then I would slip back into berating myself for being so weak and failing to handle this simple act of life that other women manage so gracefully. Rationally, I knew this was in no way my fault, but my emotions ran wild, blaming me and shaming me.

I have never had a problem talking about medical issues. I fought to have breast and testicular self-exams taught in a religious high school that argued that these were "sexual" issues and therefore inappropriate. I've always felt that treating issues related to menstruation and pregnancy and childbirth as "taboo" disempowered women, making their health issues "dirty" or "embarrassing." And I have advocated for eliminating the distinction between "mental illness" and "physical illness." I am a firm believer that mind and body are inextricably linked and that there is no such thing as "mental" illness. So it was with great humility and regret that I admit to myself that I had not spoken to anyone about my experience with postpartum depression because I felt like it was "TMI" (too much information), that somehow it was embarrassing to admit that I was being treated in a mental health facility and that I was having a "women's" problem. Until one day when one of my closest friends mentioned her postpartum depression. And I told her that I had felt the same things she did. And we looked at each other and started to weep, exclaiming in unison, "Why weren't we talking to each other!" Yes, why weren't we? We talked about everything else, and I mean everything. We could have offered each other so much support and love through this ordeal, but we didn't. Because this is the thing of which you do not speak. And that was the day that I knew I had to speak. I started to mention my postpartum depression to friends and family members when there were appropriate opportunities to do so. And more often than not, this led to crying and hugging and regretful moans of "Why didn't we talk to each other?" I felt so alone, and yet all I needed to do was to say the words "I have postpartum depression," and I would have realized that all the scary things I was going through were not unique. I had an entire sisterhood who knew my pain, and I knew theirs. But we all felt shamed into silence.

CAITLYN, TWENTY-FOUR YEARS OLD

Ever since I was a teenager I looked forward to being a mother. The idea of another human being needing me more than anything else in the world gave me a feeling I cannot even begin to put into words. It was something that I continued to dream about and had a strong desire for. I pictured myself having at least two children but was open to maybe having three, if it felt right.

Although my husband and I were not married at the time, in October 2014 we found out that I was pregnant and we were thrilled. My husband was actually the one who convinced me to take a pregnancy test. It definitely caught me off guard. I wanted to tell my mom in person, but I am terrible at keeping secrets, so, believe it or not, I ended up telling her via text message. Not exactly how I imagined telling my mom she was getting promoted to grandmother, but it was a weight lifted off my shoulders. We were engaged at the time, so we crammed the rest of our wedding planning into about a month, pulled some strings, and had the wedding as soon as we could so that I could still fit into my dress.

The night before my first ultrasound felt charged and exciting like Christmas Eve. I was eager, but also had my concerns. Anxieties. I am the kind of person who always thinks of the worst-case scenarios. Ever since I was a little girl I would worry about things that were illogical or impractical for me to be worried about, but they somehow dominated my thoughts nonetheless. As I got older I noticed this problem getting worse. For example, I would constantly be afraid of my loved ones getting into a car accident, and I was terrified of my house burning down. I know that it likely sounds silly, because these were things I could not control. Of course, these were reasonable things to be worried about, but not so much that they controlled daily thoughts, as they did. Naturally, because of my tendency to overthink, as excited as I was for my ultrasound, I could not help but worry about receiving bad news. My heart pounded on the way to the doctor, and it beat harder and harder, filling up my ears, all the way up until I was lying down on the examination table in the ultrasound room. The screen was turned on, and I could barely believe my eyes. My little inch-long baby was squiggling around on screen. Although my little nugget was only about an inch long and the size of a pecan (according to one of my many pregnancy apps, of course), everything was already perfect.

I always wanted to have a little boy first. I am not quite sure why, but I wanted to have a boy first and then a girl second, if I could have designed it. This feeling changed once I was pregnant. Right from the moment I found out I was pregnant I had this instinctual feeling that the baby was a girl. I only thought of girl names, and in my mind it was not even an option for the baby to be a boy. My husband was away for work when I had my twenty-week ultrasound, when they reveal the gender of the baby, so my mom came to the appointment with me. I had the ultrasound technician write down the gender and put it in a sealed envelope instead of telling us right away. The envelope was given right to a baker, and they were going to make the inside of a cake either blue or pink. A few days later our closest family and friends gathered for our gender reveal party. My husband and I cut into the cake, and as soon as I saw pink I jumped for joy and cried tears of pure happiness. That day will always be one of the best days of my life. Pink icing and my dreams were becoming a reality.

The remainder of my pregnancy went very smoothly. I was tired most of the time and had some heartburn, but that was the extent of any unpleasant symptoms. Pregnancy felt natural to me, so I was already thinking about my next little bundle of joy. Surprisingly, my anxiety and depression were at an all-time low during my pregnancy. I was previously on antidepressants, but when I found out I was expecting my doctor recommended that I stop my medication if I could. I was weaned off of it, and I surprisingly felt great.

As my due date approached, I was anxious to meet my baby girl. The due date came and went. At this point I was extremely uncomfortable and barely sleeping at night. I did everything I could to try to naturally induce labor on my own. I ate spicy foods, inhaled a ton of pineapple, walked laps around the mall, you name it. I was feeling a lot of pressure from my uterus onto my pelvis but not even a slight contraction. It was at this point in my pregnancy that it was decided by my doctor and I that my best option at that point was to medically induce labor. Although I was disappointed I didn't get to experience going into labor on my own, as I had always expected, it was surreal knowing that I knew the date that I would finally meet my baby. My husband and I spent the night in the hospital, and the idea that I was going to meet my little girl soon was pure bliss. I had my makeup and hair done in anticipation of photos after her birth. I figured that since I had such a smooth pregnancy the labor would be a breeze, too. Spoiler alert: I was wrong.

The painful contractions started fast and gave me little break in between. As my contractions got more intense, I had the anesthesiologist give me an epidural. I wanted to kiss the anesthesiologist when he walked in the room, as I saw him as the physical embodiment of pain relief. The epidural went well, and I was out of pain and comfortable again before I knew it. Despite the strong contractions, I was dilating very slowly, only about a centimeter every two hours. The wait was brutal. Finally, after an agonizing several hours, I was seven centimeters dilated when my epidural began to stop working—it simply wore off—and I felt everything again. The doctors could not seem to figure out why I was no longer responding to the medicine. They almost did not believe me when I told them it had worn away. The anesthesiologist came in to do another epidural, which helped, but I was still in an incredible amount of pain. After twenty-four hours of being in the hospital I was finally ten centimeters dilated. It was, blessedly, time to push! Yet after close to two hours of pushing there was still no baby. I was frustrated that my body wasn't doing what it was supposed to do. I was discouraged and disappointed. I began to develop a fever and my blood pressure began to elevate, so the doctors decided to prep me for a cesarean section, to ensure that the baby and I would both remain healthy. I did not expect to have a cesarean, but I will admit that I did breathe a sigh of relief knowing that it was almost over. As I lay on the operating table I finally heard my little girl cry and it was the best sound that I have ever heard. Welcome to the world, Vivian Rose. Our daughter was born on June 17, at 10:51 p.m. She weighed eight pounds, nine ounces and was twenty-one inches long. I thought that the hard part was over, but, sadly, little did I know that it had only just begun.

They brought me into the recovery room, where I was finally able to meet my daughter. I had a short period of bliss, but it was not long after that when I began to hemorrhage and the extreme blood loss caused me to lose consciousness. I was trying to communicate, but the lack of oxygen to my brain made it impossible for me to control the words that were coming out of my mouth. My uterus would not contract as it was meant to, causing me to lose massive amounts of blood. They tried massaging my uterus (which is extremely painful) and gave me multiple blood transfusions. I wish now that I could say that I do not remember any of this, but I will painfully admit that I do and that I remember a lot. I remember being scared and not knowing what was going to happen. At 4 a.m., only about five hours after giving birth, my vitals were so unstable that the doctors really began to worry. I had lost so much blood and they still could not get the bleeding to stop. They decided to open me up again, by entering back in through my recent cesarean incision, to see if they could get the bleeding to stop that way. I was so incoherent at this point that my poor husband had to sign a consent form to perform a hysterectomy. That was their only option, as they could not risk letting me bleed much longer. In order to save my life, they would need to take out my uterus.

I woke up the next morning and was told what had been done. Initially, I was just happy to be alive with my healthy baby girl. I was in the intensive care unit, and at first I was told that I would not be able to see my daughter until I was back up in the maternity unit. They did not want to bring a newborn baby to the area of the hospital where the patients are the sickest. This broke my heart. Thankfully, I had a wonderful lactation nurse who demanded that I be able to see my daughter, and so I was able to get my hands on my daughter so that I could breastfeed. Unfortunately, I was too weak, and after a few days of trying I was told my body was too focused on replenishing itself with blood that my milk supply was pushed to second priority. My milk would not come in. This was also devastating news, an additional blow, because I so badly wanted to nurse my baby. Everything was just snowballing. Yes, I had a healthy baby girl, but I had lost so much. At the age of twenty-three, a hysterectomy had never even been a thought in my mind and I could not believe what had happened. After having spent so much of my life worrying about possible tragedies, I was ill prepared for what would actually happen to me.

My perfect labor wasn't so perfect, but my little girl is. As I said, I had always thought that I would have two or three children, and it breaks my heart knowing I will not be able to carry another baby in my belly. It was hard welcoming new life into the world and grieving the loss of my uterus at the same time. I have faith and I am sure that it all happened for a reason, but I am still searching for that reason. It does not make sense. Even though I had never thought about adoption in the past, I am excited to see what the future holds. Maybe we will expand our family through adoption or another unknown avenue, or maybe my little girl will be our one and only.

I had a lot of guilt thinking that I did something wrong with my body to make it turn against me. I remained as positive as possible through the whole ordeal, and after a week of being in the hospital I was just happy when we finally returned home.

It has been a struggle knowing I am unable to carry another baby. Although I am doing well today, waves of sadness come and go, especially when I see a new pregnancy announced on social media or among my group of friends. Please understand and do not get me wrong: I am so, so happy for all the moms out there who are about to welcome an amazing new life into the world, but I cannot help but to think about the fact that that will never be me again. It took a while for my feelings about the hysterectomy to sink in. I am still digesting this. I tried my best to put my brave face on for my family. At times, I have felt very alone because I did not have anyone to talk to who could relate to me. My biggest mistake was that I did not seek help as soon as I got home. With my history of depression I should have immediately seen a therapist or my doctor. I was having a hard time handling a newborn and dealing with all of my emotions. I felt as if I had no reason to be sad, and I felt ashamed that I was feeling so down in the dumps. I had survived a very scary experience and my little girl is as healthy as could be. What would I have to be sad about? The truth is, sometimes your emotions cannot be controlled. Your brain is a powerful thing, and when you let that "dark cloud" linger above your head for too long, everything will just pile up until you explode. There is nothing embarrassing or shameful in having issues with postpartum depression. I am thankful that my family was so supportive and they pushed me to take care of myself. The truth is I could not be a good mother until I was emotionally well.

When my daughter was about three months old, I put my pride aside and went to see my doctor. I got myself and my emotions figured out, not only for me but also for my baby. Even though I am in a better mental state now than I was a year ago, I still have bad days. I have come to accept that having bad days every once in a while is normal. Our bad days make us appreciate our good days. My little girl and I are both thriving now, and seeing her run around is still too good to be true. The most powerful thing is knowing that I am not alone; you are not alone. There are women out there who feel the same way that you do. Many women. Reaching out to other moms has been such a positive experience for me. Any woman who feels down after a negative birthing experience knows that things do get better one day at a time and you never have to suffer alone.

NANCY, FIFTY-FOUR YEARS OLD

I can still remember seeing the words "Mother suffering from postpartum depression" indelibly written into my daughter's medical records. I remember feeling shame and embarrassment—would these fateful words follow her for the rest of her life? Would every subsequent pediatrician see this, and would they judge me as a "bad" mother?

To provide a bit of context, I became a mom at twenty-two years old. Not the norm for an Ivy League–educated young woman. I had graduated college months before, and there was nothing more that I wanted than to become a mom. Graduate school and future jobs would wait—my true calling, from the bottom of my heart, was to be a mother.

My husband and I (yes, I was married, and yes, the pregnancy was planned) decided that we could handle the juggling act of him finishing graduate school and having a newborn at the same time. It did not matter that we were far away from our families and support system. We both hailed from Philadelphia and were studying in Cambridge, Massachusetts. It did not matter that our college and law school friends thought we were crazy; they just did not understand. Truthfully, I am not sure that we understood; we had no idea what it meant to have a baby—especially since we were only babies ourselves.

Nevertheless, we found ourselves pregnant three months after I graduated from college. I had suffered a miscarriage earlier that year, and I was determined to get pregnant that summer. The miscarriage had left some scars, buried just below the surface, and the anxiety soared when I started bleeding with this second pregnancy. Though my scars were emotional, I worried about my physical ability to bear a healthy child. Would I have another "mis"? Was there something wrong with me? I was given progesterone and told to stay in bed for those precarious first three months, and so I did exactly that. I was going to do this right.

Finally, I entered my second trimester and received the "all clear." Despite reassurance from my doctor and the fact that my pregnancy was progressing both normally and obviously, somehow, my anxiety never really abated, and I remember rubbing my ever-growing belly continuously all day, willing the baby to move. In fact, I was convinced that I was making the baby move and, by doing so, I was assuring myself that all was really OK. Every time that I felt a flutter or a kick, I could breathe again, until the anxiety crept in once more. I remember my mother looking at my maternity tops—in those days we wore flowing muumuu blouses to accentuate our bellies—and commenting that the fabric was literally worn out from my constant massaging. It was almost compulsive, and my only way to feel some semblance of control.

Because this was the mid-1980s, I did not even know the sex of my growing baby. We did not get ultrasounds or blood tests that would show the crucial, defining parts of the baby's anatomy. Secretly, I hoped for a girl, but I convinced myself that it was a boy. I spent my whole life trying to protect a person whom I did not know at all.

The rest of the pregnancy went smoothly—the only notable fact was the constant chocolate craving that lasted for the remaining six months. I recall one trip to the market, and the clerk smiling as I loaded Oreos, chocolate milk, brownie mix, and M&Ms onto the counter. And that was for just my midday snack! I had a real thing for chocolate treats and rubbing a hole in my maternity shirts.

I became more excited, and nervous, as my due date approached. I was convinced that I would go into labor early, so eager to meet my baby, and I think that I willed my baby to arrive five days before my due date. Once my baby decided that the moment had arrived to come into the world, the kid wasted no time: we arrived at the hospital at 8 p.m. and my daughter was born before midnight. No time for epidurals or any of the other fun stuff. I endured a few hours of hard and fast natural childbirth, motivated by sheer will and the intense desire to meet my "meant to be." I will never forget the moment when they put my rose-lipped, beautiful baby girl on my tummy—surely life was now perfect!

"We get to plan a wedding," I said to my husband, as I looked up at him, tears in my eyes. I had my little girl. She was healthy. I could see her move, and I could massage her little back on the outside now. She was my dream come true.

From the moment she was born it was all-consuming. "It" being a euphemism for motherhood. My love for my daughter was profound, but also intense, and we had a symbiotic, interdependent relationship, just as we had when she was inside of my womb. She liked to be stimulated constantly, and when I left her for our first date night at four weeks old she cried the entire time that we were apart. We needed one another, had separation anxiety during the rare moments when I was doing something away from her, and my life was no longer my own. Instead of wearing holes in my maternity shirts, I wore paths in the Cambridge roads, as we walked and walked and walked, spending our days outside, walking around the campuses and parks and shops. I now realize that this was my defense mechanism and that my walking was a way to distract myself from ruminating, worrying, and feeling blue. Though my mother and other members of our family would visit us to help, I spent most of my time alone with my daughter. My husband graduated law school less than two months after our daughter was born, and he then spent all of his time studying for the bar exam.

By the time we reached her eight-week checkup, with a kind and gentle pediatrician who had come highly recommended to us, I was well known in the office. I had established a rapport with the staff and, perhaps, an identity for myself with the staff. I was the famous (infamous) mother who called the day after we got home from the hospital to ask the nurse if I was correct in waking up my newborn daughter several times during the night to nurse. I assumed that every mom had to wake up their sleeping babies to eat—wasn't that how it worked? Weren't those "sleepless nights" the common woes that had everyone complaining? The notorious perils of new motherhood? The nurse put me on hold that first morning and asked me to repeat the question to others in the office: Was I really waking up my daughter? Did she gain weight in the hospital? Were her diapers wet? Yes and yes, I answered demurely. The nurse was kind, and I remember her reply: "Never wake up a sleeping baby. You don't know how good you have it."

And I did have it good. My daughter was a wonderful baby. Clearly we had no issue bonding. She really did, remarkably, sleep through the night from day one. She nursed easily and gained weight regularly. I was still navigating through the brand new, unknown territory of motherhood, but we were finding our groove. Until our extended family—particularly my in-laws—arrived to celebrate my husband's graduation. I could not wait to introduce the group to our daughter. Our amazing, beautiful, sleeping, nursing daughter.

If I had to pinpoint a tipping point, this visit was it. This is when the trouble really started. And it started as abruptly as when they all walked into our tiny apartment and proceeded to tell me everything that I was doing wrong. Or, more accurately, that everything that I was doing was wrong.

"Don't burp the baby like that," they chastised. "Don't put her down on her side or back. You are holding her the wrong way!"

At that moment, it was like a switch was flipped. Just like that, every feeling of confidence that I had built fell away, and every suppressed bit of anxiety soared to the surface. In my life—for my whole life—I was used to doing everything well. If I am being totally honest, I would say that I was always trying to be "perfect," and after their criticism, I felt as though I was a failure. There was no middle ground. I went from our cozy routine and enchanting bond to being scared to even hold my own daughter. I was convinced that I was a horrible mother. My life's dream was a nightmare. I would escape to the shower and sob as the water cascaded down my face. I would find my hands shaking as my fears grew and multiplied.

My husband was wonderful. He encouraged me and supported me as best as he could, but I am not sure that he could understand the feeling of being absolutely overwhelmed and terrified by our gorgeous, cooing baby. Doubts ruminated through my head; it was like I was stuck on a carousel of negativity. How would I get through each day? What else am I doing wrong? How do people have more than one baby? Will this get better and will I ever feel like myself again?

And so, we ended up at the pediatrician's office for our daughter's checkup, and the tears just flowed. He scribbled "mother" and "postpartum depression" on her chart and reassured me that my daughter was doing beautifully. He told me "this will pass" and smiled like a friendly conspirator to my husband.

I am not sure that either of these well-meaning men could truly grasp the palpable anxiety and indescribable fear that took over during that time. It was so real that it felt like an actual lead weight in my chest. Surely my hormones were responsible for a great deal, and the "well-meaning" (or just "mean") family members were like gasoline to the flickering embers of anxiety.

The weeks went by, and I started to feel a bit better each day. It took time and patience, and mistakes and tears, and I am not sure if I ever fully "got over it." But I got through it, and that stage did pass. I think of this time often. Over three decades later, I can still feel the anguish and can remember the feeling of the shower water mixing with my tears as they poured, like a deluge, over my cheeks. I can still remember the shame at getting my diagnosis of "postpartum depression" on my daughter's records. All of this time has passed, but the emotions are still visceral and real.

I am still working on bettering myself and finding strength in my inner voice and mom gut, drowning out external negativity. I put effort into not listening to the criticism of others, and I am still dealing with hormones that can create palpable anxiety at certain times. Over thirty years ago my daughter and I got into our own rhythm, and we both learned to navigate a world filled with uncertainties. My second daughter was born three years later and, fortunately, I did not experience these same feelings of depression after her birth.

But I will never forget these moments or the lessons learned. I still worry about my daughter, I still love her, and there are times when it is as if I am wearing a proverbial hole in my muumuu, willing her to move when she is struggling or in her own time of crisis.

But, most of all, I will never again be embarrassed by being less than perfect. I know that I have done the best I can, which is pretty darn great—and done well by her, for myself, and as a mother. I have lived up to what I was always meant to be. And now, I have no doubt about it.

STEFF, THIRTY-THREE YEARS OLD

Maybe I should have known when I took the pregnancy test.

Or maybe I should have guessed it when I would wake up in drenching night sweats during my pregnancy with Grace, after having yet another nightmare of miscarrying.

Perhaps an alarm should have gone off when I had that one, recurring thought, stuck on repeat in my mind, of my Grace dying during my scheduled C-section.

Maybe it was clear when I asked my husband, John, if our baby was OK within seconds of him meeting her.

That was after the countless times that I almost asked the nurse for her to be on a heart monitor or if she was healthy.

I think that I finally knew for sure when I found myself waking up approximately 2,941,946 times a night to make sure that my baby wasn't dead, because I had absolutely convinced myself, for no actual reason, that she was going to die of sudden infant death syndrome (SIDS) in her sleep.

Truth be told, yes, I still wake up every night with the panic. At least twice a night I still check on Grace to make sure that she is still breathing. It has been almost ten months.

In the state of New Jersey, where I live, you fill out a questionnaire to determine your "at-risk-ness" for postpartum depression. I remember filling it out after my first child, my beloved son, Jackson, was born. The survey asked something like "Are you anxious?"

"Um, my kid just left the NICU and is being treated for a virus that I never heard of before that happened to have tried to kill him so, yeah, I would say yes. I am *anxious*."

"Do you cry?" Yes. See above.

For Grace, though, I had no reason to be anxious. She was not in the neonatal intensive care unit (NICU) or fighting some terrifying illness. I had no reason to cry. She was not my first baby, nor was she struggling. But I was. And I did. Not often, but I did enough to know that something was not right. I was not myself.

So, I did what any normal mom would do: I kept it inside, assuming that it was like a cold. It would go away with liquids and time and "rest."

It didn't.

Instead of going with my gut and addressing the problem head-on, I found roundabout ways to figure out the source of my plight. I got my thyroid checked. I was born with congenital hypothyroidism; that diagnosis means that I was born without a thyroid. When your thyroid is messed up, it can lead to depression, so I had my levels checked. They were fine.

Except I was not. I was not fine in any way. Eventually, I made an appointment with my OBGYN, and we talked about my state and the feelings that I was having. And I talked to John. I opened up to him by letting him know that I didn't feel like "me"—and that I was really anxious and that I felt like I might need some help. Of course, he was incredibly supportive.

So, at my visit to my OBGYN we had a lovely talk about postpartum depression and her own "breaking point." She shared with me that there was a time in her own life when she knew that something just was not right. As a survivor of postpartum depression herself, she has been able to provide incredible support, and just knowing that she had been through it helped me to look at myself more closely, recognize the signs, and stop treating it like a virus that would go away in a week or two.

And then, a few nights later, I had my own breaking point.

I woke up in the middle of the night to make sure that Grace was breathing. My nightly ritual. She had spit up earlier in the evening, and she was swaddled and was sleeping contentedly, soundly, and happily. My brain told me, "Oh, good, you should be sleeping, too!" but my heart would *not* let me. And my stomach turned into knots and I went kind of nuts. All of a sudden, my mind was racing with thoughts. They were all over the place, including, "Wait. What did you do when your friend was drunk in college? You didn't let them sleep on their back because remember? Yes. They could choke on their vomit. And, shit, Grace spit up earlier today!"

"Are you an idiot?" I asked myself, admonishingly. "You are going to kill Grace. She is going to spit up and she is going to choke and die and you are going to wake up in the morning and boom. She is going to be dead. Get her elevated."

Consumed by these thoughts, I then started pacing. And staring. And crying.

After an eternity, I calmed down a bit—at least enough so that tears went away. But John woke up, and he asked me why I was up.

The words came out like my own spit-up.

"Grace is going to die if I don't get her elevated, and I cannot find anything to make her bassinet elevated, so I am just going to sit here and watch her sleep. I am nervous that she is going to spit up again."

John stayed calm. For both of us. He picked up a small pile of folded laundry and he put it under the bassinet to elevate it. The gesture took merely two seconds, an action that was obvious with a clear head to employ.

And once Grace's head was elevated, I slept more soundly than I had in months. Years, maybe.

The next morning, in the light of day, John asked me when I was going to start seeing someone about my anxiety.

And so I did.

I was in weekly therapy sessions from the time Grace was eight weeks old until the time she turned one. It was incredibly helpful and wonderful. It was salient for me to have that time—an hour that I could cherish—to myself and to be "selfish" and to talk about anything and everything that is going on in my mind and my heart and my feelings on different things. All of the things. But, more than just taking this me time, I must emphasize what has been the most beneficial: having found the right therapist. And oh my goodness, for my counselor, for this woman, I have no words. She is that good. Truth be told, I know that I basically paid her to be nice to me, but I love her. And she got me. I needed that.

So yes, I have come very far from my place at the bottom, but every once in a while some feelings come back. When they come back, though, they hide in feelings of social anxiety or through really interesting fears that I never had before, like large crowds or fearing that my husband is hurt. Anxiety is something that morphs and changes, and we have to learn to evolve with it.

I know that this anxiety is going to be an ongoing issue for me, and that I have to constantly keep myself in check. I have accepted it within myself that I will, undoubtedly, be back in therapy at some point in my life. But, more important, I know that I deserve the therapy.

As a new mom, or even as a veteran mom, society makes us feel that we have to be this perfect woman with small thighs, a creative mind, a clean house, well-behaved children, and perfect makeup who makes dinner each night. It's not like that. It's scary and hard and frustrating and amazing and perfect and overwhelming and the most difficult thing I have ever done.

My children are the most important part of my life. But they're not my entire life. I deserve happiness and joy and comfort and relaxation. I deserve to have my thoughts heard and to keep myself in check.

But, as a new mom, or a mom of Irish twins, I do implore you to do the following: please keep in touch with yourself. Check in with yourself to see if you feel like you. And note if you feel like "not you." Don't feel guilty for having thoughts that carousel through your brain that have no business being there. You should know that it is normal. And it is OK. But talk them out. Talk them through. Work on them. Write them out. Sing them out. Find a counselor or therapist. Get help. It is so most definitely worth the copay. Pinky promise. Because you are worth it.

10

❖ ❖

Hope

"How are you doing?"
    "Are you feeling better?"
  "Why aren't you working?"
  "Are you still getting help?"
  People ask me these questions—among others—every day.
  I understand the questions. I know that they come from care and concern, and I appreciate the compassion from the people around me: friends, family members, readers, and people on the street who stop me as I go about my days.
  Now that I am post-postpartum, I have started a new phase of life. In many ways it is a great one.
  My kids make my heart sing. Belle is amazing. By that I mean that she fits the dictionary definition of the word, truly, as she causes great surprise or wonder—astonishing. She and I are so similar, and our deep bond allows us to have deep talks. We talk about a lot of things; it is like having a conversation with an adult, and a bright one at that. It is awesome. And yes, by that I mean extremely good—excellent.
  This past spring, as I drove her home from a long day at school, we had a conversation about babies. I asked her, lightheartedly, if she would still want to use a baby name that we had talked about for another baby, if we were to have one.
  "I am not sure," she started.

I watched her body, her shoulders held high. I saw her face, which is like looking into my own, and I saw her brain working from behind her little glasses.

"You already have your fruit, Mom."

"What?" I asked her. I didn't get what she meant, at first, though somewhere, deep inside, I think I may have; I think I was just incredulous—awed.

"You are a tree, Mommy. You made two pieces of fruit. You made my brother and me. And that is the fruit that your tree is supposed to make."

And just like that, I started to sob. And it wasn't because I was sad; it was because I was moved. And, amazingly, I did not have to tell her that.

"I know that you are crying happy, Mama," and she smiled at me as I turned my head around to her while stopped at a red light.

More recently, Belle's big mind in her little body made magic once again, bringing me to my knees. I received an e-mail from her first-grade teacher with the subject line "This WILL make your day."

That, in itself, is a wonderful line of text to receive and, of course, I was eager to read his message. I figured that she had given him a big hug and perhaps said something particularly sweet that day in school.

But that is not what the body of his e-mail said. His message was long, effusive, and genuine: "This is something I had to share with you, given it was one of those moments that left me speechless and with chills."

Her teacher had read a book to the class called *The Lion Inside*, written by Rachel Bright and illustrated by Jim Field. It teaches, as the e-mail explained to me, that everyone has both a "mouse" and a "lion" inside at all times; the moral of the story instills confidence in children, as it illustrates that we all have many feelings all at once, and that that is OK—that we all feel nervous sometimes and bold at others.

After they finished reading the book, the class had a discussion about its theme, and just as they were preparing to transition to their next activity, my little girl raised her hand.

When she was called on, she stood up. She stood up with confidence and conviction and said, boldly, "Fear is just a reason to try harder."

And her class clapped for her, her teacher beamed with pride. When I read this e-mail, I cried. First, I was so touched by her teacher's kindness and the support that he gives to her and to our family. But, more than anything else, I was astounded by my daughter's wisdom.

Fear is just a reason to try harder.

My daughter has fears. She comes by this honestly. Some of her fears are from hard life experience (she has been brought up with a family that is bursting with love, but also brimming with some hard stuff), and some are from small moments that impacted her (like when seagulls attacked her food at the beach when she was two, so now she avoids all flying creatures). I often feel guilty that she has the burden of anxiety, as she must have been impacted by our "hard story" over the past few years since her brother was born.

And she must see it. There are so many times in my life when, as much as I hate to admit this, my fears rule me. Fear is prohibitive for many, and I am often among that group.

I get nervous to advocate for myself, or to write about a controversial topic or to get on an airplane. I get scared to share my story, because I am scared that I will be judged—that the stigma of mental health issues will overshadow all that is good about me and I will be branded with a scarlet "S" for "sufferer," and then it will all be over for me.

But Belle reminded me that I cannot continue to let fear get in my way. Never, not ever.

Fear is just another reason to try harder.

I will keep on working hard. I will keep on hugging my daughter and getting that extra love. And I will keep on sharing who I am in an effort to help others.

I will face my fears, because my daughter showed me that fear is something to run toward and not away from. Belle is my greatest inspiration and my most amusing muse.

And then there is my second child. My Beau. While Belle changed my life by making me a mother, Beau changed me deeply, making me into the woman I am today. Despite a difficult start, he has taught me about resilience and strength. He has taught me how to love fiercely and unconditionally. He has taught me that life does not ever really look like how you had planned for it to look, and sometimes, if you are lucky, the new picture is the most beautiful picture imaginable. He is naughty, strong willed, sweet, funny, and smart, all in a thirty-two-pound, strawberry blonde, blue-eyed package.

He loves the things that he loves in a way that only he can. These things include his big sister, bacon, and the cream inside of Oreo cookies. If I tell him to put his glasses back on, and he is feeling particularly rebellious, he will put them on his face upside down. If I tell him to stay in his room, Beau will fall asleep at the threshold where his wall-to-wall carpet meets the hardwood of the hallway. He toes the line, and I love it. I love that he rebels, because I think that he will continue to fight for the things that he wants and in which he believes.

Besides being strong willed, Beau is empathetic. He cries if his big sister cries. He asks, over and over, to make sure that the people he loves are happy. If they are not, you can see the pain on his face. He is filled with love, and he is filled with spunk. I love him more than I can ever express. For as many words as I know, I do not have the words to explain my intense gratitude for this little boy.

My children are now actual people, and they have become best friends. They choose to sleep together every night. They have dozens of games that they have made up, the rules that only they know. They hold each other closely in the night. Despite their age difference, they are two sides of the same shiny, crazy, silly, lovely, dancing coin. Sometimes I look at them and I feel completely—well—complete.

My daughter is extraordinary. Her brilliance astounds me.

My son is remarkable. His strength humbles me.

I know that our family is exactly as it should be, and I feel so blessed for the two miracles that I have the pleasure of calling ours.

And then, other times, it still hurts.

Mourning the loss of that other life, the one that I once imagined, is much easier as I watch Belle and Beau play together, making up their games, giggling with identical laughs, and I can actually feel intense joy in these precious moments. I feel it more profoundly than others feel anything on this earth, I imagine. And, at the same time, it is also hard.

It is my juggling act. It is hard for me to explain what it is like to walk the line that I do each day.

On one hand, I am functional. I get out of bed each morning, even though some days, for a myriad of reasons, it is harder or easier than others. I take care of my children. I pack them lunches with notes. I dress them in cute outfits, and 72 percent of the time they agree to wear them. I make dinners. I invent recipes.

I work very hard. I write every day. I write my blog. I freelance for other publications. I respond to e-mails of readers who are looking for help—to feel less alone. I record a podcast. I get interviewed for television and magazines and other websites. I share my story, trying to scream about things that other people will only talk about in a whisper.

I am continuing to fortify my tribe. I spend time with friends. I connect over the phone and through text messages every single day. I make lunch dates and chai dates and cocktails with spicy peppers and tequila, and I so cherish these times.

I decorate my home, I do my best to pick out cute outfits, I shop for shoes online, and I try to make family traditions that are unique to us.

And, on the other hand, I am a mess.

On this other, less beautiful hand, I am not OK. I do not always sleep very well. I do not always eat very well. I go to at least four different therapy appointments each week. I see a therapist, a couple's therapist, a psychiatrist, and a dietician, at minimum. I struggle, at times, even just for a moment, every single day.

And the hardest part of all is that I do not know how to be both things, and so I walk the line.

I share just enough good and just enough not-so-good. I *live* some really good and some really bad. I think, in our own ways, we all do.

Lately, more than ever, I have been acutely aware that I am balancing on a strange tightrope in my life. Juggling. Tightropes. I am the star of my own cirque de mommay.

Almost every day, in so many different situations, I must walk the line. There are the obvious times, with things that all parents face. I want to raise good, strong people. My children are old enough, now, to recognize that actions have consequences. I do not want them to make excuses or to be disingenuous—with themselves or others—but, like everything else, this is a balance. Do I want my children to be earth-shatteringly upset if (and when) they slip up? Of course not. We all need to have perspective. But I also want them to know what it means to be accountable, to have grace.

One of the hardest lines to walk is with regard to my health. I do not want my daughter to worry about me or for my already anxious child to be *more* anxious or for my own struggles to make her feel like she has to take care of me. Or for her to think that my size is normal. And these desires are in conflict.

I am raising a daughter and a son in an age when eating disorders are an epidemic, and even in my own family they are exposed to a lot of chatter about weight, food, size, skinny, and fat.

And then there is the whole honesty thing. I teach my children to tell the truth. Honesty is the most salient value to me. And I think that I may tell my children more than the average parent because of this. For instance, if I am having a fight with a family member and my daughter overhears, when she asks what is going on, even if I initially try to do so, I cannot lie. I try to say, "Oh, it was someone you don't know," but then, inevitably, I fold. What I end up saying is "I was having a little argument with my mom, but you know that everyone has arguments sometimes. We love each other very much so we both get sensitive. We will always love each other. We made up. You have nothing to worry about." And that is the truth. And perhaps that is too burdensome for my little humans, but in my mind I am showing her that problems can exist *and* be fixed *and* that we will always love her *and* that nothing could ever change that. There is no manual for this parenting thing. I am just doing my best. And they show that to me each day. I must be doing at least something right.

And I get to say that they came from my tree. They are the sweetest pieces of fruit that I could ever imagine.

It only helps that my marriage is stronger than ever, and that is because of, and not in spite of, all of the hard work that it took for us to get here. We cherish our family, enjoy our friends, and have found a new normal.

There is so much good.

And, as there always is with life, we have struggles.

"How are you doing?"

"Are you feeling better?"

"Why aren't you working?"

"Are you still getting help?"

The questions.

Here are the answers, though I think that you know them already.

I am doing fine. Some days are better than others. Some days I am energetic and confident, and I hit the ground running. Nothing can stop me. Other days it is hard to get out of bed. Not dramatically hard, as it used to be, but it can be harder than it should be. I am feeling better emotionally, a lot of the time, but also working extremely hard in therapy to fix some of the underlying issues that caused me to suffer as I have. I can now see how far I have come, and I am so thankful that I got the treatment that I have received. Without professional help, I would not be here today.

My work may not be what it was before, but I am working harder than ever. I am working at being a strong woman, a devoted mother, a present wife, and an advocate for mental health. I am working on being a good person.

Sometimes I feel haunted by old ghosts. I have triggers: songs come on the radio, smells waft through the air, the leaves turn colors, and I remember the last time, that fall three years ago, that I actually felt like my old self. I am not that woman anymore. And that is a good thing.

I am a tree.

Some days I feel pretty, with colorful leaves. Some days I provide shade or comfort. Some days I look worn and bare, and I feel cold and frail.

But I am a tree, still standing, strong and mighty, with deep roots, growing taller as I go.

I am a tree. I grow babies. I grow dreams.

And, most of all, I grow hope.

Notes

1. Amy Wenzel, *The Oxford Handbook of Perinatal Psychology* (Oxford: Oxford University Press, 2016).

2. Wenzel, *The Oxford Handbook of Perinatal Psychology.*

3. K. A. Yonkers, K. L. Wisner, D. E. Stewart, T. F. Oberlander, D. L. Dell, N. Stotland, C. Lockwood, et al., "The Management of Depression during Pregnancy: A Report from the American Psychiatric Association and the American College of Obstetricians and Gynecologists," *Obstetrics and Gynecology* 114, no. 3 (2009): 703–13, doi.org/10.1097/AOG.0b013e3181ba0632.

4. Yonkers et al., "The Management of Depression during Pregnancy."

5. Yonkers et al., "The Management of Depression during Pregnancy."

6. Yonkers et al., "The Management of Depression during Pregnancy."

7. Marie-Paule Austin, Lucy Tully, and Gordon Parker, "Examining the Relationship between Antenatal Anxiety and Postnatal Depression," *Journal of Affective Disorders* 101, no. 1–3 (2007): 169–74, doi:10.1016/j.jad.2006.11.015.

8. Gemma L. Gladstone, Gordon B. Parker, Philip B. Mitchell, Gin S. Malhi, Kay A. Wilhelm, and Marie-Paule Austin, "A Brief Measure of Worry Severity (BMWS): Personality and Clinical Correlates of Severe Worriers," *Journal of Anxiety Disorders* 19, no. 8 (2005): 877–92, doi:10.1016/j.janxdis.2004.11.003.

9. G. J. Diefenbach, D. F. Tolin, S. A. Meunier, and C. M. Gilliam, "Assessment of Anxiety in Older Home Care Recipients," *Gerontologist* 49, no. 2 (2009): 141–53, doi:10.1093/geront/gnp019.

10. Austin, Tully, and Parker, "Examining the Relationship between Antenatal Anxiety and Postnatal Depression."

11. Christine Dunkel Schetter and Lynlee Tanner, "Anxiety, Depression and Stress in Pregnancy," *Current Opinion in Psychiatry* 25, no. 2 (2012): 141–48, doi:10.1097/yco.0b013e3283503680.

Bibliography

Austin, Marie-Paule, Lucy Tully, and Gordon Parker. "Examining the Relationship between Antenatal Anxiety and Postnatal Depression." *Journal of Affective Disorders* 101, no. 1–3 (2007): 169–74. doi:10.1016/j.jad.2006.11.015.

Diefenbach, G. J., D. F. Tolin, S. A. Meunier, and C. M. Gilliam. "Assessment of Anxiety in Older Home Care Recipients." *Gerontologist* 49, no. 2 (2009): 141–53. doi:10.1093/geront/gnp019.

Gladstone, Gemma L., Gordon B. Parker, Philip B. Mitchell, Gin S. Malhi, Kay A. Wilhelm, and Marie-Paule Austin. "A Brief Measure of Worry Severity (BMWS): Personality and Clinical Correlates of Severe Worriers." *Journal of Anxiety Disorders* 19, no. 8 (2005): 877–92. doi:10.1016/j.janxdis.2004.11.003.

Kendall-Tackett, Kathleen A. *Depression in New Mothers: Causes, Consequences, and Treatment Alternatives.* 2nd ed. London: Routledge, Taylor & Francis Group, 2010.

Miller, Laura J., and Elizabeth M. Larusso. "Preventing Postpartum Depression." *Psychiatric Clinics of North America* 34, no. 1 (2011): 53–65. doi:10.1016/j .psc.2010.11.010.

Schetter, Christine Dunkel, and Lynlee Tanner. "Anxiety, Depression and Stress in Pregnancy." *Current Opinion in Psychiatry* 25, no. 2 (2012): 141–48. doi:10.1097/yco.0b013e3283503680.

Sockol, Laura E., C. Neill Epperson, and Jacques P. Barber. "Preventing Postpartum Depression: A Meta-Analytic Review." *Clinical Psychology Review* 33, no. 8 (October 21, 2013): 1205–17. doi:10.1016/j.cpr.2013.10.004.

Wenzel, Amy. *Coping with Infertility, Miscarriage, and Neonatal Loss: Finding Perspective and Creating Meaning.* Washington, DC: American Psychological Association, 2015.

Wenzel, Amy. *The Oxford Handbook of Perinatal Psychology.* 1st ed. Oxford: Oxford University Press, 2016.

Yonkers, K. A., K. L. Wisner, D. E. Stewart, T. F. Oberlander, D. L. Dell, N. Stotland, C. Lockwood, et al. "The Management of Depression during Pregnancy: A Report from the American Psychiatric Association and the American College of Obstetricians and Gynecologists." *Obstetrics and Gynecology* 114, no. 3 (2009): 703–13. doi.org/10.1097/AOG.0b013e3181ba0632.

Index

delivery: first, 19–21; second, 50–51

depression: characteristics of, 78–79; in pregnant women generally, 25, 27, 30–31; prenatal anxiety as predictor of, 31. *See also* prenatal distress

detachment. *See* numbness of feelings during pregnancy

dilation of cervix. *See* cervical dilation

distress. *See* fetal distress; prenatal distress

effacement. *See* cervical dilation

emergency room (ER): with second child, 1, 71–73; during second pregnancy, 40–41

emotional support, 92

epidural, 49, 50

expectations, rigid, 79, 80

fertility issues, 9

fetal distress, 15–18

fetal heart monitor, 16, 17–18

generalized anxiety disorder (GAD), 31, 60

grief, 74–78, 128

history, mother's mental health, 28, 56

hope, 125–31

inducing labor, 12, 18

informational support, 92

intolerance of uncertainty, 79

intrusive thoughts, 29, 57

labor and delivery: first pregnancy, 10–21; inducing labor, 12, 18; preparation for, 10; second pregnancy, 46–51

love story, 5–8, 87–91

medical treatments for prenatal distress. *See* antidepressant and anti-anxiety medications

menstrual cycle and mother's mental health history, 28

mental health history, mother's, 28, 56

migraine, 45–46

mood changes in pregnant women, 26

mood stabilizers, 73. *See also* antidepressant and anti-anxiety medications

morality bias, 79

nausea during pregnancy, 26–27, 37, 43

negative social support, setting boundaries against, 92–94

numbness of feelings during pregnancy, 41, 43–45, 46

obsessive compulsive disorder (OCD), 56–57, 61–62, 79

overestimation of responsibility, 79

pain management during labor and delivery, 19, 50

Panettiere, Hayden, 87–88, 90

panic disorder, 25, 60

perfectionism, 79

perinatal distress. *See* prenatal distress; postpartum depression; recovery from perinatal distress

perinatal distress, stories: Amie, 98–107; Caitlyn, 112–16; Erica, 107–11; Nancy, 116–21; Steff, 121–24

physical changes during pregnancy, 26

positive-negative-positive sandwich, 93

postpartum depression: characteristics of, 78–79; differences from general depression, 79; impact on marriages, 88; *postpartum period* defined, 78; prenatal anxiety as predictor of, 31; risk factors for, 31, 79; supporting sufferers of, 80–81, 92

postpartum depression, author's experience of: beginning, 63–66; hospitalization, 68, 72–73; impact on marriage, 87–91; initial therapy, 65; life after, 125–31; official diagnoses, 73; reluctance to take medication, 65; self-harm, 66–67; treatment, 73–74

postpartum psychosis, 57, 109–10

About the Author

Rebecca Fox Starr is a writer, blogger, podcaster, and mental health advocate with an unyielding desire to help other mental health sufferers. Among her greatest accomplishments, Rebecca has used the success of her blog, *Mommy, Ever After*, to create a private, online forum for women in which they are able to open up about psychological and social issues that they would otherwise be too afraid to address. Her story has been featured in the *New York Times*, on ABC News, and in all forms of media across the world. Rebecca lives and writes with her husband, children, and Yorkie in the suburbs of Philadelphia. The *Mommy, Ever After* blog can be found at www.MommyEverAfter.com.